People experience life through frameworks of meaning they create for themselves—both singly and collectively. With this fundamental postulate, Jonathan D. Raskin lucidly, comprehensively, and sometimes irreverently cuts through the fog of abstraction that often obscures the genuinely novel and exciting contributions a constructive approach makes to the practice of psychotherapy. Synthesizing developments in personal constructivism, coherence theory, social constructionism, narrative therapy, and contextual approaches, this deceptively compact and engagingly readable book invites the reader to imagine how a vast range of human struggles can be dissolved in a heartbeat through a shift of stance or framing. Dozens of diverse case vignettes vividly conjure the transformative power of language and relationship to challenge and change how clients configure their worlds and, with this, themselves. I recommend this volume to all therapists yearning to infuse new vision into their work by experimenting with the principles and procedures of *Constructive Psychotherapies*.

—**Robert A. Neimeyer, PhD,** coeditor, *Journal of Constructivist Psychology;* Director, Portland Institute for Loss and Transition, Portland, OR

Dr. Raskin has succeeded where many others have failed. He has given constructive psychotherapy a clear, vibrant, contemporary voice. In lucid prose, with the use of helpful case examples, Raskin crystallizes how constructive theory and practice combine to simplify and amplify the work of today's clinicians. Others who have attempted this feat have either drifted into abstract philosophy or provided a reductionistic list of disconnected clinical suggestions. For my money, Raskin's eminently readable narrative provides the coherent guide for which we have long been waiting.

—**Jay Efran, PhD,** Professor Emeritus of Psychology, Temple University, Philadelphia, PA

Constructive Psychotherapies

Theories of Psychotherapy Series

Acceptance and Commitment Therapy
  Steven C. Hayes and Jason Lillis

Adlerian Psychotherapy
  Jon Carlson and Matt Englar-Carlson

The Basics of Psychotherapy: An Introduction to Theory and Practice, Second Edition
  Bruce E. Wampold

Behavior Therapy
  Martin M. Antony and Lizabeth Roemer

Brief Dynamic Therapy, Second Edition
  Hanna Levenson

Career Counseling, Second Edition
  Mark L. Savickas

Cognitive–Behavioral Therapy, Second Edition
  Michelle G. Craske

Cognitive Therapy
  Keith S. Dobson

Constructive Psychotherapies
  Jonathan D. Raskin

Dialectical Behavior Therapy
  Alexander L. Chapman and Katherine L. Dixon-Gordon

Emotion-Focused Therapy, Revised Edition
  Leslie S. Greenberg

Existential–Humanistic Therapy, Second Edition
  Kirk J. Schneider and Orah T. Krug

Eye Movement Desensitization and Reprocessing (EMDR) Therapy
  Mark C. Russell and Francine Shapiro

Family Therapy
  William J. Doherty and Susan H. McDaniel

Feminist Therapy, Second Edition
  Laura S. Brown

Gestalt Therapy
  Gordon Wheeler and Lena Axelsson

Interpersonal Psychotherapy
  Ellen Frank and Jessica C. Levenson

Multicultural Therapy: A Practice Imperative
  Melba J. T. Vasquez and Josephine D. Johnson

Narrative Therapy, Second Edition
  Stephen Madigan

Person-Centered Psychotherapies
  David J. Cain

Psychoanalysis and Psychoanalytic Therapies, Second Edition
  Jeremy D. Safran and Jennifer Hunter

Psychotherapy Case Formulation
  Tracy D. Eells

Psychotherapy Integration
  George Stricker

Rational Emotive Behavior Therapy, Second Edition
  Albert Ellis and Debbie Joffe Ellis

Reality Therapy
  Robert E. Wubbolding

Relational–Cultural Therapy, Third Edition
  Judith V. Jordan

Solution-Focused Therapy
  John J. Murphy

Theories of Psychotherapy Series
Matt Englar-Carlson, Series Editor

Constructive Psychotherapies

Jonathan D. Raskin

 AMERICAN PSYCHOLOGICAL ASSOCIATION

Copyright © 2025 by the American Psychological Association. All rights, including for text and data mining, AI training, and similar technologies, are reserved. Except as permitted under the United States Copyright Act of 1976, no part of this publication may be reproduced or distributed in any form or by any means, including, but not limited to, the process of scanning and digitization, or stored in a database or retrieval system, without the prior written permission of the publisher.

The opinions and statements published are those of the Author, and do not necessarily represent the policies of the American Psychological Association. The information contained in this work does not constitute personalized therapeutic advice. Users seeking medical advice, diagnoses, or treatment should consult a medical professional or health care provider. The Author has worked to ensure that all information in this book is accurate at the time of publication and consistent with general mental health care standards.

Published by
American Psychological Association
750 First Street, NE
Washington, DC 20002
https://www.apa.org

Order Department
https://www.apa.org/pubs/books
order@apa.org

Typeset in Minion by Circle Graphics, Inc., Reisterstown, MD

Printer: Gasch Printing, Odenton, MD
Cover Designer: Beth Schlenoff Design, Bethesda, MD
Cover Art: *Lily Rising*, 2005, oil and mixed media on panel in craquelure frame, by Betsy Bauer

Library of Congress Cataloging-in-Publication Data

CIP Data has been applied for.
Library of Congress Control Number: 2025009411

ISBN 9781433839955 (paperback)
ISBN 9781433839962 (epub)
ISBN 9781433849183 (pdf)

https://doi.org/10.1037/0000468-000

Printed in the United States of America

10 9 8 7 6 5 4 3 2 1

Dedicated to the memory of Franz Epting (1937–2023),
my advisor, mentor, and friend;
and to Franz's husband, Mark Eliot Paris (1957–2024),
who exemplified strength in the face of adversity.
They are deeply missed.

Contents

Series Preface	*xi*
How to Use This Book With APA Psychotherapy Videos	*xvii*
Acknowledgments	*xix*
1. Introduction	3
2. History	9
3. Theory	21
4. The Therapy Process	35
5. Evaluation	91
6. Future Directions	103
7. Summary	111
Glossary of Key Terms	117
Suggested Readings and Resources	125
References	129
Index	151
About the Author	159
About the Series Editor	161

Series Preface

Matt Englar-Carlson

Some might argue that in the contemporary clinical practice of psychotherapy, the focus on evidence-based intervention and effective outcomes has overshadowed theory in importance. Maybe. But, at the same time, psychotherapists adopt and practice according to one theory or another because their experience, and decades of empirical evidence, suggests that having a sound theory of psychotherapy leads to greater therapeutic success. Theory is fundamental in guiding psychotherapists in understanding why people behave, think, and feel in certain ways, and it provides the guidance to then contemplate what a client can do to instigate meaningful change. Beyond this, theory ensures a consistent, structured, and ethical approach to therapy, informs treatment planning, and empowers clients by providing tools and rationale they can apply outside of sessions. It also enhances therapists' self-awareness and aligns their practices with established standards, supporting both professional and personal growth. Still, the role of theory in the helping process itself can be hard to explain. This narrative about solving problems may help convey theory's importance:

> Aesop tells the fable of the sun and wind having a contest to decide who was the most powerful. From above the earth, they spotted a person walking down the street, and the wind bet it could get the person's coat off. The sun agreed to the contest. The wind blew fiercely, but the person clutched their coat tightly. The harder the wind blew,

the tighter the person held on. Then it was the sun's turn. Focusing all its energy on creating warm, gentle sunshine, the sun eventually caused the person to remove the coat.

What does a competition between the sun and the wind to remove a person's coat have to do with theories of psychotherapy? This deceptively simple story highlights the importance of theory as the precursor to any effective intervention—and hence to a favorable outcome. Without a guiding theory, a psychotherapist might treat the symptom without understanding the role of the individual. Or we might create power conflicts with our clients and not understand that, at times, indirect means of helping (sunshine) are often as effective—if not more so—than direct ones (wind). In the absence of theory, a psychotherapist might lose track of the treatment rationale and instead get caught up in social correctness and not wanting to do something that looks too elementary.

What exactly is theory? The *APA Dictionary of Psychology* defines *theory* as "a principle or body of interrelated principles that purports to explain or predict a number of interrelated phenomena" (American Psychological Association, n.d.). In psychotherapy, a theory is a set of principles used to explain human thought and behavior, including what causes people to change. In practice, a theory frames the goals of therapy and specifies how to pursue them. Jay Haley (1997) noted that a theory of psychotherapy ought to be simple enough for the average psychotherapist to understand but comprehensive enough to account for a wide range of eventualities. Furthermore, a theory guides action toward successful outcomes while generating hope in both the psychotherapist and client that recovery is possible.

Theory is the compass that allows psychotherapists to navigate the vast territory of clinical practice. Just as navigational tools adapt to advances in thinking and expanding territories, theories of psychotherapy evolve to incorporate breakthroughs in science and technology while also responding to societal changes and cultural shifts. The different schools of theories are commonly referred to as waves—for example, the first wave of psychodynamic theories (e.g., Adlerian, psychoanalytic), the second wave of learning theories (e.g., behavioral, cognitive behavioral), the third wave of humanistic theories (e.g., person-centered, gestalt, existential), the fourth wave of feminist and multicultural theories, and the fifth wave of postmodern and constructivist theories (e.g., narrative, solution-focused, constructivist). In many ways, these waves represent how psychotherapy has adapted and responded to changes in psychology, society, and epistemology as well as to changes within psychotherapy itself. The wide variety of theories highlights the diverse ways human behavior can be conceptualized depending on the lens through which it is viewed (Frew & Spiegler, 2012). However, established theories of psychotherapy are increasingly challenged to decenter dominant ways of thinking and being that are rooted in a Western worldview. This shift calls for a realignment of psychotherapy that serves a broader and more culturally diverse population, emphasizing inclusivity and accessibility alongside clinical effectiveness. Theories and psychotherapists must move beyond an exclusive focus on individualism and individual change, incorporating community action, social justice, and an understanding of systemic inequities. Expanding psychotherapy to be more inclusive of marginalized and under-resourced populations also requires addressing barriers that make it inaccessible to those outside of wealthier demographics. By integrating these perspectives, psychotherapy and the theories that guide it can remain dynamic and responsive to the complexity of the world and the full range of human experiences that accounts for a client's context and intersectional identity (American Psychological Association, 2017).

It is with these two concepts in mind—the central importance of theory and the natural evolution of theoretical thinking—that the *APA Theories of Psychotherapy Series* was developed. This series was created by my father (Jon Carlson) and myself. Though educated in different eras, we both had a love of theory and often spent time discussing the range of complex ideas that drove each model. Even though my father identified strongly as an Adlerian and I was parented and raised from the Adlerian perspective, my father always espoused an appreciation for other theories and theorists—and that is something I picked up from him. As university faculty members teaching courses on the theories of psychotherapy, we wanted to create learning materials that not only highlighted the essence of the major theories for professionals and professionals in training, but also clearly brought the reader up to date on the status of the models focusing on future directions with an emphasis on the inclusive application of the theories with clients representing the range of identities. Often in textbooks on theory, the biography of the original theorist overshadows the evolution of the model. In contrast, our intent was to highlight the contemporary application of the theories as well as their history and context—past, present, and future.

As this project began, we faced two immediate decisions: which theories to address and who best to present them. We assessed graduate-level theories of psychotherapy courses to see which theories are being taught, and explored popular scholarly books, articles, and conferences to determine which theories draw the most interest. We then developed a dream list of authors from among the best minds in contemporary theoretical practice. To that end, authors in the series are the leading proponents of that approach as well as knowledgeable practitioners. We asked authors to review the core constructs of the theory, bring the theory into the modern sphere of clinical practice by looking at it through a context of evidence-based practice as applied to clients with intersectional identities, and clearly illustrate how the theory looks in application.

There are nearly 30 titles in the series, with many titles now in their second or third editions. Each title can stand alone or can be put together with a few other titles to create materials for an advanced course in psychotherapy theories. This option allows instructors to create a course featuring the approaches they believe are the most salient today. To support this end, APA Books has also developed multiple videos for most of the approaches that demonstrate the theory in practice with clients. Many of the videos show psychotherapy over six sessions with the same client, while others focused on theory-specific case conceptualization. Consult APA Books for a complete list of available video programs (https://www.apa.org/pubs/videos).

We live in a time where it appears that the facts of the world associated with events are increasingly under debate. Some might wonder how one person could experience an event in such different ways or how the framing of an event can evolve over time as public perception is manipulated to serve other interests. *Constructive Psychotherapies* gets right at the root of these questions as it explores how individuals and groups construct, create, and interpret their personal realities, emphasizing the subjective and evolving nature of personal meaning rather than objective truths. It asks how clients construct their experiences and identities, encouraging them to explore and revise these constructs to foster personal growth and change. In *Constructive Psychotherapies*, Jonathan D. Raskin gives the reader an illustration of how our experiential realities are constituted as much or more by the stories we construct and share than by the cold hard facts of our surroundings. These constructed meanings yield and affect experiential realities that impact mental health and how people experience their lives and relationships. Raskin shares a range of clinical examples that shows how constructive psychotherapy encourages a dialogue that respects multiple perspectives while fostering critical reflection and understanding to explore the subjective interpretations and narratives people create around their experiences. This therapeutic conversation helps clients create new possibilities for understanding themselves and their situations, ultimately leading to personal growth and change. Raskin has created a monograph that will truly make the reader think about how one thinks, and that process itself can be freeing and illuminating in many ways.

REFERENCES

American Psychological Association. (n.d.). Theory. In *APA dictionary of psychology*. Retrieved January 17, 2024, from https://dictionary.apa.org/theory

American Psychological Association. (2017). *Multicultural guidelines: An ecological approach to context, identity, and intersectionality*. Retrieved January 17, 2024, from https://www.apa.org/about/policy/multicultural-guidelines.pdf

Frew, J., & Spiegler, M. (2012). *Contemporary psychotherapies for a diverse world* (1st rev. ed.). Routledge.

Haley, J. (1997). *Leaving home: The therapy of disturbed young people*. Routledge.

How to Use This Book With APA Psychotherapy Videos

Each book in the Theories of Psychotherapy Series is specifically paired with a video that demonstrates the theory applied in actual therapy with a real client. Many videos feature the author of the book as the guest therapist, allowing students to see an eminent scholar and practitioner putting the theory they write about into action. The video programs have a number of features that make them excellent tools for learning more about theoretical concepts:

- Many video programs contain six full sessions of psychotherapy over time, giving viewers a chance to see how clients respond to the application of the theory over the course of several sessions.
- Each program has a brief introductory discussion recapping the basic features of the theory behind the approach demonstrated. This allows viewers to review the key aspects of the approach about which they have just read.
- The videos feature volunteer clients in unedited psychotherapy sessions. This provides a unique opportunity to get a sense of the look and feel of real psychotherapy, something that written case examples and transcripts sometimes cannot convey.

The books and videos together make a powerful teaching tool for showing how theoretical principles affect practice. In the case of this book, the video *Constructive Therapy in Practice*, which features Jonathan D. Raskin as the guest expert, provides a vivid example of how this approach looks in practice. For more information, please visit APA Videos (https://www.apa.org/pubs/videos/).

Acknowledgments

Writing a brief book on psychotherapy is difficult! I wish to thank Susan Reynolds at the American Psychological Association and the "Theories of Psychotherapy" series editor, Matt Englar-Carlson, for their patient support. I am also extremely grateful to my development editor, Molly Gage, for attentively guiding me through the revision process; her input helped strengthen the manuscript.

I owe a debt of gratitude to constructive colleagues both living and deceased who have greatly influenced me—including Sara Bridges, Vivien Burr, Trevor Butt, Gabriele Chiari, Rue Cromwell, Don Domenici, Valerie Domenici, Ken Gergen, Don Granvold, Stephanie Lewis Harter, Richard Hayes, Larry Leitner, Michael Mahoney, Sheila McNamee, Spencer McWilliams, Bob Neimeyer, Greg Neimeyer, Amberly Panepinto, Mark Paris, Harry Procter, Kenneth Sewell, Caroline Stanley, Bill Warren, and David Winter. I am especially grateful to two mentors and friends: my late doctoral advisor, Franz Epting, who introduced me to the world of personal construct psychology and constructive therapies, then served as a kind and dedicated mentor for 3 decades; and Jay Efran, whose seminal influence has shaped not only this volume and how I conduct psychotherapy but more broadly how I approach life. Franz and Jay have helped transform my construct system!

On the family front, thanks to my parents, Paula and Sherman, for their ongoing support and care, as well as to my brother Daniel, my sister-in-law Kayoko, my nephew Taro, and my partner's daughter, Evelyn. Further thanks to Tessa, my incredibly loving partner, for her endless patience and kindness; I could not succeed without her.

Finally, thanks to my two daughters, Ari and Noa. Ari's forthrightness, determination, and self-confidence are qualities I strive to emulate, while I am forever humbled by Noa's astounding sensitivity and insight. My conversations with Noa about her experiences as a budding therapist reminded me what it is like being new to the field, which helped enormously in writing this book.

Constructive
Psychotherapies

1

Introduction

Homo sapiens is the species that invents symbols in which to invest passion and authority, then forgets that symbols are inventions.
—Joyce Carol Oates, "The Calendar's New Clothes"

This provocative quote succinctly captures the spirit of constructive therapies. Oates's words remind us that people construct the realities they experience as much as (or more than) they discover them. Constructive therapies, the focus of this book, invite clients to reflexively examine the accounts they have built for themselves—and to entertain new ones when existing accounts back them into a corner. Although thinking constructively potentially opens possibilities, it can also be unsettling because it violates the traditional assumption that experience corresponds to (and is the direct product of) external reality. The outside world is highly salient to people; therefore, their role in making sense of it typically goes

https://doi.org/10.1037/0000468-001
Constructive Psychotherapies, by J. D. Raskin
Copyright © 2025 by the American Psychological Association. All rights reserved.

unnoticed. This may explain why human meanings—despite their constructed nature—are not easily trifled with. Because people experience their constructions of the world as real and stable, they cannot simply discard or ignore them: "The way an event is construed and *narratized* becomes virtually inseparable from how it is experienced" (Efran et al., 1990, p. 110).

Consequently, constructive approaches to therapy can initially seem counterintuitive because what people experience often seems directly imposed by an impartial reality, not something they play a role in creating. Yet, in many instances, the constructed "made-upness" of it all seems commonsensical, even obvious. For example, although red traffic lights mean "stop" and green ones mean "go," there is nothing inherent in those colors that makes this so (Cameron, 2020; Cutolo, 2023). Red and green have been assigned these meanings by human beings. Different designations could just as easily be made. Sticking with colors, pink is commonly associated with girls, and blue with boys. Why? Because people decided this. However, this was not always so. Before World War I, babies were generally dressed in white (Cahn, 2024). The associations of specific colors with gender did not develop until later—and have not always been what they are today. Until the 1940s, pink was for boys, and blue for girls (Cahn, 2024)!

Although their assignment to stoplights and babies' clothes is a human invention, the red, green, pink, and blue colors themselves must be "true" in a way that goes beyond human invention, right? Not necessarily. Returning to stoplights, Japanese stoplights use what many people would identify as blue rather than green. This is because in Japanese culture, green (*midori*) is considered a specific type of blue (*ao*) rather than a stand-alone color (Spektor, 2023). The implication here is that we individually and culturally sort visual experiences into color categories. These categories are influenced but not determined by wavelengths of light. The structure of our eyes and brains is equally or more important in determining what we see.

The human eye's three photoreceptors for color vision can only register blue, green, and red light (Hussey et al., 2022). However, the same is not so for vision across all species. The eyes of birds (and maybe reptiles and fish) have an additional photoreceptor that registers ultraviolet light, which people cannot see. Thus, birds "experience a world awash in extra colors humans can't imagine" (Fox, 2020, para. 3). These additional colors do not simply make the world prettier for our avian friends. They make it easier for them to spot food, aiding their survival (Fox, 2020). Critically, the color categories various animal species use to divvy up the world reflect the exigencies of their perceptual experience, not a literal reproduction of reality itself. The acronym ROYGBIV (red, orange, yellow, green, blue, indigo, violet) was not discovered in an attic trunk. People made it up because it helped them usefully account for their experience. If birds could talk, they would catalog and label colors quite differently.

Even gender and sex, ideas that seem disinterestedly imposed by the world, might best be viewed as humanly invented templates for organizing experience. In many cultures, the idea that there are two genders is increasingly being challenged—but not just by transgender and nonbinary folks who reject traditional gender distinctions. It is also being contested by scientists, who are realizing that both sex and gender are more complicated than the either/or distinctions that people generally make (Ainsworth & Nature Magazine, 2018; Thomson, 2023; Wilchins, 2004). Gender roles, although influenced by biological differences, are underdetermined by them. As a case in point, economics research has found that in societies in which agriculture historically relied on plow farming (which requires upper body strength), people developed more rigid and less equal gender norms; a strict division of labor evolved in which biological male individuals plowed the fields, whereas biological female individuals handled domestic chores (Alesina et al., 2013). However, in societies in which the plow was not predominant, more flexible gender roles emerged. In other words, notions of gender originate as much from the social and cultural practices people devise as they do from biology.

The constructed nature of sex and gender extends beyond economics and culture into those "hard science" disciplines in which human understandings are commonly viewed as mirrors of (rather than constructions of) reality. Yet, even here, we create as much as we discover—and then, as Joyce Carol Oates reminded us, we reify our invented accounts. To wit, sex is not as firm an attribute of the external world as we often believe. As many as 5% of animal species can change sex (Thomson, 2023). Worms and snails, for instance, have both male and female sex characteristics, whereas various types of frogs, reptiles, and fish change sexes over the course of their lifetimes (Thomson, 2023). Even in mammals, sex can be fluid. For instance, biological research has suggested that the gonads of mice "teeter" between male and female across their lifespans and must be constantly "maintained" (Ainsworth & Nature Magazine, 2018). With all due apologies to Mickey and Minnie Mouse, the firm male–female dichotomy we have created does not always withstand scrutiny. And things are no clearer in humans than mice. Various forms of atypical human development call into question our notions of sex as an unarguable binary. For example, people we traditionally assume are "truly" male (because they have XY chromosomes) can develop female genitalia if they are insensitive to the male sex hormone androgen (Ainsworth & Nature Magazine, 2018). Taken-for-granted ideas of "male" and "female" are imperfect human accounts that we often mistake for truth itself.

FROM CONSTRUCTIVE THEORIES TO CONSTRUCTIVE THERAPIES

All this suggests that experiential realities are constituted as much or more by the stories people construct and share than by the cold hard facts of their surroundings. Such sentiments reflect the broad contours of *constructive theories*, which contend that people and the social groups they form know the world indirectly through mental templates of their own creation (Burr, 2025; Gergen, 2015; Glasersfeld, 1995; Kelly, 1955a, 1955b; Lyddon, 1995; Raskin, 2002). Although constructive ideas can be found in many disciplines, they have been applied in psychology to areas ranging from perception to personality to education (Kelly, 1955a, 1955b; Maturana & Varela, 1992; Steffe & Kieren, 1994). This book asks: What can constructive theories offer to psychotherapists? Therapists who fall under the constructive moniker are curious about how constructed meanings yield and affect experiential realities. *Constructive therapies*, therefore, disrupt and reinterpret clients' reified meanings and thereby initiate reconstruction processes that open new possibilities.

This volume introduces you to constructive therapies. These therapies emerged from the proposition that people, alone and in concert with one another, *construct* meaningful understandings of the world, which they use to make sense of their surroundings. Generally, this works seamlessly—so well, mind you, that people regularly mistake their constructions for reality itself. For instance, Sherry[1] blames her relationship difficulties on "daddy issues," Joaquin attributes his anger outbursts to "impulse control problems," and Maria insists her career difficulties are the result of "low self-esteem." Using these terms to make sense of experience is not inherently problematic, but when Sherry, Joaquin, and Maria start reifying "daddy issues," "impulse control problems," and "low self-esteem," respectively, as fundamental truths rather than handy but imperfect human accounts, they can become imprisoned by them. In other words, because the invented nature of our descriptions is so often forgotten or overlooked, we easily find ourselves ensnared in conundrums of our own making. Confusing our constructions with reality is often at the root of mental distress. As philosopher and scientist Alfred Korzybski (1994) famously observed, "A map *is not* the territory" (p. 750). In a nutshell, constructive therapies highlight the human tendency to conflate our linguistic and conceptual maps with the territory. They remind us that we are all cartographers and, in so doing, they conceive of therapy as a process to help clients revise and update their maps so that they will be more useful.

A NOTE ON TERMINOLOGY

In keeping with the work of Mahoney (1988, 2003) and Hoyt (1994, 1996), the broader and more inclusive term *constructive therapies* is used throughout this book as opposed to the term *constructivist therapies*. This accounts for the diverse perspectives under the constructive banner that go by different names, including *constructivist, social constructionist, narrative,*

---

[1] All cases in this volume use pseudonyms. Client identifying details have also been disguised.

and *postmodern* (Efran et al., 2014; Neimeyer & Mahoney, 1995; Neimeyer & Raskin, 2000; Raskin, 2002; Shotter, 1995). Technically, *constructivism* focuses more on individual meaning-making, whereas *social constructionism* emphasizes social, relational, and collaborative constructive processes. However, in everyday practice, the constructivist–constructionist distinction is often blurry. Therefore, using the term *constructive therapies* allows us to playfully mix and match constructivist and constructionist ideas. Additionally—and just as importantly—it also lets us emphasize the complementary dual definitions of the word *constructive*, which means both "to build up" and "serving a useful purpose" (Google, n.d.). These two definitions wonderfully convey the pragmatic and meaning-focused clinical strategies and techniques discussed throughout this volume.

2

History

Constructivism is a perennial in the history of ideas.
—Michael J. Mahoney (2003, p. 212)

Constructive ideas are not new. They can be found throughout history, even if they have often been unfairly disparaged or disregarded (Glasersfeld, 1995). Historically, those espousing a constructive orientation encountered trouble gaining traction for their viewpoint because "by renouncing the quest for certain knowledge about reality, they had deprived themselves of the very argument philosophers use to distinguish knowledge from mere opinion or belief" (Glasersfeld, 1995, p. 25). It is difficult to defend a constructive stance because "the traditional way of thinking was (and still is) far too strong to be shaken" and critics usually demand that one do so on realist (not constructive) grounds (Glasersfeld, 1995, p. 25).

Nonetheless, over the past 100 years or so, constructive perspectives have garnered increased attention and established more of a foothold.

ANCIENT GREECE AND CHINA

Ancient Greek pre-Socratic thinkers offered the earliest philosophical observations anticipating modern constructive psychologies. For instance, in the late 6th and early 5th centuries B.C.E., the Greek skeptic Xenophanes mused about the impossibility of knowing reality beyond our human constructions of it:

> Yet the true and known—at least in respect of non-evident things—no human being knows; for even if by chance he should hit upon it, still he knows not that he has hit upon it but imagines and opines. (Xenophanes, as cited in Lesher, 1978, pp. 1–2)

Roughly a century later, the Sophist philosopher Gorgias expressed a similar sentiment (Higgins, n.d.). He suggested that "things don't exist in the way we perceive them" and that "even if they did we have no way to know if they do, and even if we knew we could not communicate that knowledge directly to others" (McWilliams, 2022, p. 448). Gorgias's fellow Sophist Protagoras put it more succinctly when he famously observed that "man is the measure of all things" (Bonazzi, 2020, para. 1). Xenophanes's, Gorgias's, and Protagoras's statements effectively capture the constructive view of knowledge as personal and private rather than an exact duplicate of the world it presumably represents (Salas Llanas, 2018).

The related notion that the knowledge we build continually changes with experience can be traced not just to other pre-Socratic Greek thinkers like Heraclitus (who famously said that we never step in the same river twice) but also to ancient 6th and 5th century B.C.E. Chinese thinkers, such as Lao Tzu and Buddha (with their emphasis on the impermanence of experience; Graham, 2019; Mahoney, 2003; McWilliams, 2016b). Buddhism's discouragement of attachments "to viewpoints, obsessions, constructions, and preferences" (McWilliams, 2016b, p. 440) presages later constructive psychologists, such as George Kelly (1955a, 1955b), who warned against reifying ideas and believed that all theories (including his own) were eventual candidates for the trash bin. Thus, the notion that we construct and perpetually revise accounts of the world was evident from early in human history.

LOCKE, BERKELEY, AND HUME

Empirical philosophies hold that we know the world via our senses—and modern science, which took its cue from empirical philosophies, therefore privileges observation and measurement. To the "hard-nosed empiricist," sensory information is the basis of experimental evidence and is often assumed to reflect "the character or state of an observer-independent world" (Glasersfeld, 1995, p. 31). However, Ernst von Glasersfeld (1995), a founder of radical constructivism (described later in this chapter), challenged strictly realist interpretations of empiricism, pointing to constructive themes in the works of empiricists John Locke, George Berkeley, and David Hume—none of whom, in Glasersfeld's view, "was so naïve a realist" that they believed "experimental evidence provides data that reflects the character of the state of an observer-independent real world" (Glasersfeld, 1995, p. 31). For instance, although John Locke (1690/2019) embraced a more passive view of mind compared with later constructive thinkers, his concept of "reflection" retained a place for constructing ideas—meaning that he was not as wedded to the "blank slate" view of mind as usually assumed (Glasersfeld, 1995). Instead, Locke attributed human knowing not just to sensory experience but also to the mind reflecting on its own processes. He stated that "all ideas come from sensation or reflection" (Locke, 1690/2019, p. 78).

Anglo-Irish Bishop George Berkeley took things even further, confusing many philosophers with his famous statement *esse est percipi* ("to be is to be perceived"). This phrase expresses Berkeley's (1710/2009) philosophical idealism in which he holds that things only exist when perceived by the mind. From a constructive viewpoint, Berkeley was suggesting that through our own mental construction processes, we bring the experiential world we know into being (Glasersfeld, 1992/2007). Consistent with this, Berkeley challenged Locke's (1690/2019) belief that *primary qualities* (e.g., size, shape, number, motion, time) are more objective, real, and less dependent on the observer than *secondary qualities* (e.g., taste, smell, color). Berkeley countered that primary qualities like time and motion are "generated by the experiencing subject" and imposed on successive experiences (Glasersfeld, 1995, p. 34). Accepting Berkeley's interpretation

> wipes out the major rational grounds for the belief that human knowledge could represent a reality that is independent of human experience. For if extension, motion, time, and causation are dependent on the reflective activity of a subject, one cannot describe in human terms what "reality" would be like *before* it is experienced. (Glasersfeld, 1995, p. 34)

Like Berkeley, David Hume also saw a role for the mind, which he felt creates associations between ideas. Hume (1977/2006) proposed three ways the mind does this through distinguishing (a) *resemblance* (identifying ideas that are similar), (b) *contiguity* (identifying ideas that are close together in time and space), and (c) *cause and effect relationships* (identifying consistently observed relationships between contiguous events, then making a connection between them such that the first is believed to result in the second). Importantly, even though the mind makes associations among ideas, one can never be certain that the presumed events they refer to are connected beyond our having linked them: "When we say, therefore, that one object is connected with another, we mean only that they have acquired a connexion in our thought" (Hume, 1777/2006, Part II, para. 3). These connections, which are perceptions of the mind, are all we know: "The mind has never anything present to it but the perceptions, and cannot possibly reach any experience of their connexion with objects" (Hume, 1777/2006, Part 1, para. 12).

VICO, KANT, AND VAIHINGER

The Italian philosopher Giambattista Vico offered one of the first fully constructive theories of knowledge (Gash & Glasersfeld, 1978). He posited that *verum esse isum factum* ("truth itself is made"), noting that "the world of civil society has certainly been made by men, and . . . its principles are therefore to be found within the modifications of our own human mind" (Vico, 1744/1948, p. 85). To Vico, "everything we experience is initially a personal construction" (Gash & Glasersfeld, 1978, p. 26). This is reflected in his statement that "to know (*sciere*) is to put together the elements of things" (Vico, 1710/1988, p. 46). Interestingly, he reasoned that what limits our construing is not objective reality but rather our previous construing. In other words, Vico maintained that the constraints "we encounter spring from the history of our construction, because at any moment whatever has been done limits what can be done in the future" (Glasersfeld, 1984, p. 30). The constructions we use to navigate the world constrain how we make sense of things and—as every psychotherapist is painfully aware—are not always easily revised or discarded.

Immanuel Kant's rational idealist philosophy also anticipates today's constructive psychologies (Glasersfeld, 1995, 1984). Kant (1783/2004) distinguished *phenomena* (our sensory experiences, which are all we truly know) from *noumena* (the presumed world beyond our ideas). He believed that people rationally transform phenomenal experience (which initially is a jumbled mess of sensations, what Kant referred to as the *manifold*) into constructed explanations and understandings. In other words, the mind imposes innate *categories of understanding* onto sensory experience (Kant, 1781/1990). Thus, knowledge results from the mind molding sense data into something meaningful and coherent. This way of thinking anticipates the constructive theories of personal construct psychology and radical constructivism—both of which contend that sensory information is acted on and organized by the human mind, which converts it into constructed schemas (Glasersfeld, 1995; Kelly, 1955a, 1955b). The resulting knowledge allows us to viably navigate life, even if this knowledge can never "match" the world "as is." Kant had a tremendous influence, yet his constructivism is often minimized and overlooked:

> In spite of Kant's thesis that our mind does not derive laws from nature, but imposes them on it, most scientists today still consider themselves "discoverers" who unveil nature's secrets and slowly but steadily expand the range of human knowledge. (Glasersfeld, 1984, p. 20)

Building on Kant's work, the late 19th and early 20th century German philosopher Hans Vaihinger (1911/1935) developed his "philosophy of as if" in which he proposed that people create explanatory *fictions* and then live "as if" these fictions are inarguable truths that mirror the world. As he put it, "We do not know objective reality absolutely but only infer it" (Vaihinger, 1911/1935, p. 3). Expecting criticism of this view (which persists to this day), Vaihinger articulated as effectively as anyone ever has the position that a constructive perspective does not prevent proceeding scientifically or coherently with everyday life. He held that "thought does not mirror reality and yet does arrive at reality" because "mental processes are ultimately adequate" (Vaihinger, 1911/1935, p. 140). What, according to Vaihinger, allows us to proceed?

> It is not the correspondence with an assumed "objective reality" that can never be directly accessible to us, it is not the theoretical representation of an outer world in the mirror of consciousness nor the theoretical comparison of logical products with objective things which, in our view, guarantees that thought has fulfilled its purpose; it is rather the practical test as to whether it is possible with the help of those logical products to *calculate events that occur without our intervention* and to realize our impulses appropriately in accordance with the direction of the logical structures. (Vaihinger, 1911/1935, p. 3)

Vaihinger's emphasis on the practical utility of knowledge anticipates constructive psychology's emphasis on the viability of human understandings, discussed next.

CONSTRUCTIVE THINKING IN EARLY PSYCHOLOGY

Vaihinger was a contemporary of two founding figures of modern psychology: Wilhelm Wundt and Hermann von Helmholtz—both of whom, it has been argued, were receptive to constructive themes (Glasersfeld, 1995; Mahoney, 1988, 2003; Stoll, 2020). Wundt and Helmholtz were not the only figures in the early years of professional psychology whose work encompassed constructive motifs. William James, John Dewey, Charles Pierce, and other advocates of philosophical pragmatism greatly influenced constructive psychology's emphasis on *viability* (the workability of ideas within specific contexts) over *validity* (the ability of ideas to replicate the world as it is; Butt, 2000; Menand, 2001; Paris & Epting, 2015). We may never know whether our constructed knowledge matches a presumed external world, but we determine how well it allows us to predict events and accomplish desired ends (Glasersfeld, 1984; Kelly, 1955a, 1955b).

Constructive refrains also appear in the work of many other 20th century thinkers whose seminal ideas have influenced modern psychology. We do not have space to discuss them all in detail. However, they include but are not limited to James Mark Baldwin (whose research on social development anticipated later constructive approaches), Frederick Bartlett (who proposed that memory is a reconstructive endeavor), Donald Campbell (who developed an evolutionary epistemology with constructive themes), Charles H. Cooley (whose writings about the "self" emphasized anticipating how others see us), Mary Whiton Calkins (whose personalistic introspective self-psychology has a constructive flavor), Frederick Hayek (who applied constructivist ideas to the study of economics), Konrad Lorenz (whose work on ethology has advanced constructive theories of knowledge), George Herbert Mead (whose pragmatistic philosophy has influenced constructive perspectives, especially social constructionism), Jean Piaget (who studied cognitive development using a constructivist lens), and Ferdinand de Saussure and Benjamin Whorf (who greatly shaped constructive ideas about human beings "living" in language, the notion that people's lived realities emerge from the language they use to organize and structure their experience; Efran et al., 1990; Glasersfeld, 1995; Mahoney, 1988, 2003). Constructive thought also contains echoes of Gestalt psychology (with its emphasis on the mind organizing sensory experience into coherent wholes), early cognitive psychology (to the extent that it conceptualizes schemas as mental creations), and humanistic–existential psychology (especially its focus on the creation of personal meaning; Epting & Leitner, 1992; Epting & Paris, 2006; Faulkenberry & Faulkenberry, 2006;

R. Holland, 1970; Juvova et al., 2015; Mahoney, 1988, 2003; Neimeyer & Raskin, 2001).

CONSTRUCTIVE IDEAS IN PSYCHOTHERAPY

In the clinical realm, several early therapies anticipated later constructive approaches. For instance, Adler's individual psychology advanced a goal-oriented humanistic brand of therapy that greatly influenced modern constructive therapies (Watts, 2013, 2017). Similarly, George Kelly's early efforts at role therapy eventually morphed into his constructive fixed-role therapy (Kelly, 1969a; Zelhart & Jackson, 1983). Kelly and Adler's approaches were more explicit in their constructivism, but nonconstructive cognitive and behavioral perspectives have exerted an influence on constructive therapies too (Dobson, 2001; Freeman et al., 2004)—although, importantly, constructive therapies move beyond equating cognition with thinking and viewing behavior as a passively determined response to environmental triggers (Kelly, 1969d).

Adlerian Influences

During the first 3 decades of the 20th century, Alfred Adler incorporated Vaihinger's notions of "as if" and "explanatory fictions" into his individual psychology, giving it a decidedly constructive flavor (Watts, 2013, 2017). Consistent with a constructive worldview, "Adlerian theory asserts that humans construct, manufacture, or narrativize ways of looking and experiencing the world and then take these fictions for truth" (Watts, 2017, p. 142). Adlerian theory not only anticipates constructive theories but also shares key characteristics when it comes to clinical applications. Like constructive therapies, Adlerian therapy emphasizes a respectful and collaborative therapy relationship, focuses on the future rather than the past, stresses client strengths rather than pathology, foregrounds the importance of context and social embeddedness, highlights the centrality of meaning, and espouses optimism about clients' potential for change (Watts, 2017). Given these commonalities, it comes as no surprise that some consider Adler to be one of the first modern constructive therapists (Watts, 2013, 2017).

Kelly's Role Therapy

Although he did not publish extensively about it until the 1950s, during the 1930s psychologist George Kelly pioneered role therapy, an approach that later evolved into fixed-role therapy, the only concrete therapy technique Kelly ever proposed (Zelhart & Jackson, 1983). The origins of role therapy can be traced to a traveling therapy clinic that Kelly founded and ran in Kansas during the Great Depression (Zelhart & Jackson, 1983). Kelly initially used psychoanalysis in the clinic but quickly became disenchanted with it, finding that any interpretation offered—no matter how preposterous—potentially provoked client change (Kelly, 1969a). Further, with so many clients desperate for services, Kelly did not have the time or resources for full-blown psychoanalysis.

Kelly's therapeutic improvisations—influenced by Korzybski's general semantics, Moreno's psychodrama, Dewey's pragmatism, and his own observation that proposing novel interpretations could initiate change (Butt, 2000; Kelly, 1955a, 1969a; Paris & Epting, 2015; A. E. Stewart & Barry, 1991)—led him to develop *role therapy* in which clients were asked to play a different role for several weeks to see what could be learned (Zelhart & Jackson, 1983). For instance, a shy client might be asked to play the role of someone more outspoken with the idea that doing so would open new behavioral possibilities that could generate sustainable change. Role therapy evolved into personal construct theory's fixed-role therapy and also influenced Kelly's later claim that behavior is an experiment (Kelly, 1970). Both fixed-role therapy and the notion of behavior as an experiment are discussed further in Chapter 4.

Cognitive Behavior Therapies

Given some of their shared historical antecedents, it is not surprising that constructive therapies have been both influenced by and are influencers of cognitive behavioral therapies (Dobson, 2001; Freeman et al., 2004). Constructive therapists place great value on both behavior and thinking. However, they conceptualize them differently than do their cognitive behavioral colleagues. As we shall see, appreciating these differences is important in transitioning to a constructive perspective.

Behavior as Independent Rather Than Dependent Variable

Traditional behavior therapy sees behavior as the outcome of *conditioning*, a reinforced response to an environmental stimulus (Slife et al., 1999). By contrast, constructive perspectives view behavior as a matter of choice— a way of asking (and actively testing) a question. George Kelly (1969d) explained it this way: Behavior therapists, he said, view behavior as a *dependent variable* (determined by its antecedents and consequences). Constructive therapists, on the other hand, view behavior as an *independent variable* (freely chosen to test a hypothesis). From a constructive mindset, behavior is an active and meaningful attempt to assess the utility of one's constructed beliefs as opposed to being a passive response elicited by the world.

For instance, consider the case of Charlotte, a client who seeks therapy for ongoing relationship conflicts. Charlotte's friends and family complain that she resorts to aggressive and rude verbal attacks whenever they disagree with her. Rather than viewing Charlotte's impolite and insulting behavior as a conditioned reaction to criticism, the constructive therapist interprets it as an attempt to test whether future criticism can be prevented by verbally shouting down other people. This shifts constructive therapies from instrumental (means-end) interventions, which manipulate clients into behaving as desired, toward constitutive (commitment and value-focused) interventions. In constitutive interventions, behavior is considered meaningful and intentional but also adjustable should a client wish to experiment with alternatives (Fowers, 2010). The takeaway message is that, like behaviorists, constructive clinicians place behavior front and center. However, rather than seeing behavior as an automatic response to external triggers, constructive therapists view it as an active effort to implement and evaluate personally invented understandings.

Beyond Just Thinking and Rationality

Cognitive therapies privilege thinking; they assume that it is our interpretations, rather than events themselves, that lead to psychological upset (Beck et al., 1979; Ellis & Joffe Ellis, 2019). This sounds constructive in that it distinguishes thoughts about the world from the world itself. Nonetheless, constructive therapies differ from cognitive therapies in two important ways.

First, unlike traditional cognitive therapies (e.g., Beck et al., 1979; Ellis & Joffe Ellis, 2019), constructive therapies do not equate construing with thinking (Cromwell, 2010; Kelly, 1955a). From a constructive standpoint, construing is not limited to rational information processing; it is much broader. Yes, construing includes logical and linear thought, but it also extends to nonverbal processes, such as feelings and bodily sensations. Constructive psychologist George Kelly suggested that dividing experience into "thoughts" and "feelings" was often more limiting than useful because it encourages drawing too firm a line between those categories; he preferred seeing thoughts and feelings as different aspects of construing—or, said another way, alternative ways of making meaning (Cromwell, 2010; Kelly, 1955a). Thus, classifying constructive therapies as cognitive approaches overlooks the more expansive, and less strictly "rational," way in which constructive therapists conceptualize construing.

Second, although cognitive therapists accept a distinction between the world and interpretations of that world, they remain wedded to the idea that the best way to assess construing is by determining its correspondence with reality (Velton, 2007). This perhaps explains their penchant for calling client beliefs "mistaken." Constructive therapists, by contrast, do not generally do this—not because they view one belief as just as good as another, but because they see all beliefs (even their own) as constructions of, rather than reproductions of, the world. Consequently, constructive therapists do not regard themselves as having better access to reality than their clients do. Thus, they concern themselves more with the viability than the validity of client construing (Butt, 2000; Paris & Epting, 2015). A constructive therapist may never know for sure how well a construct matches the world, but when a client reports not getting the desired results from a particular construct, it is time to entertain alternatives.

Although reality correspondence can sometimes be a useful way to evaluate construing, just as often, it has little connection to psychological well-being. Religious doctrines, spiritual beliefs, and philosophical commitments cannot be justified rationally; their factuality is highly questionable. However, they can be deeply meaningful and satisfying systems to live by. Constructive therapies challenge the assumption that alleviating mental distress is a simple matter of correcting false beliefs.

FROM HISTORICAL INFLUENCES TO MODERN THERAPIES

The idea that people know the world indirectly through accounts of their own making has percolated throughout human history. Although sometimes marginalized for challenging traditional theories of knowledge, constructive perspectives have endured. These perspectives inform the theories and therapies that subsequent chapters examine.

3

Theory

*What we make of experience constitutes the only world
we consciously live in.*
—Ernst von Glasersfeld (1995, p. 1)

The therapy strategies discussed herein primarily derive from three constructive theories: (a) personal constructivism, (b) radical constructivism, and (c) social constructionism. All three of these theories are complex and nuanced. The literature on them is far more extensive than what this volume can cover. Those interested in learning more about these theories should consult the Suggested Readings and Resources at the end of the book. The summaries that follow and the four premises of an integrated constructive approach will suffice as a brief introduction to constructive theory and its implications for therapy.

---

https://doi.org/10.1037/0000468-003
Constructive Psychotherapies, by J. D. Raskin
Copyright © 2025 by the American Psychological Association. All rights reserved.

PERSONAL CONSTRUCTIVISM

Personal constructivism (also called *personal construct psychology* or *personal construct theory*) holds that people devise private systems of psychological meanings made up of *personal constructs*, each consisting of two "poles": the first being an idea and the second being its perceived opposite (Kelly, 1955a, 1955b). People continually revise and expand their construct systems as they successively encounter new events (Kelly, 1955a, 1955b). Everyone's personal construct system is unique to them. Meaning is an individualized affair. To truly understand someone requires grasping how they construe events.

For example, Marjorie construes the opposite of "submissive" as "friendly," Roberta construes the opposite of "submissive" as "adventurous," and Fernando construes the opposite of "submissive" as "aggressive." Clearly, these three people mean different things when they describe themselves or others as "submissive." Therapists must pay attention to such differences. When clinicians take the meaning of "submissive" for granted, perhaps by assuming everyone defines its opposite as "assertive," they often exacerbate rather than alleviate client difficulties. For instance, encouraging Marjorie, Roberta, and Fernando to be less submissive is unlikely to engender greater assertiveness. Instead, it simply fosters behavior consistent with their notions of being "not submissive." Thus, Marjorie becomes more friendly, Roberta takes more risks, and Fernando lashes out at people—all very different consequences of being less submissive. Without inviting each of these three clients to articulate or reconstrue—or both—how they define "submissiveness," little in the way of predictable therapeutic progress can be expected. This highlights a central tenet of constructive therapies, namely that the meaning of language is not fixed; the words clients use carry distinctive and personalized meanings. Unless clinicians work to understand clients' unique meanings, therapy risks being unproductive or even harmful.

To reiterate, although people often use the same language to describe their experience, personal constructivism reminds us that what people mean when using particular words is very much an individual matter. Although this may seem obvious, people often disregard it, even in psychotherapy circles. In daily practice, therapists often rely on their own professional constructs—for instance, diagnoses from the American Psychiatric Association's (2022) *Diagnostic and Statistical Manual of Mental Disorders* (*DSM-5-TR*)—rather than the personal constructs of their clients. Although professional constructs have their place, grasping the idiographic meanings of each client is critically important to constructive therapists in planning effective and appropriate clinical interventions. In personal construct therapy, one size does not fit all. Encouraging the client with a "passive versus aggressive" construct to be less passive might be clinically productive for some but not others (Faidley & Leitner, 1993). Therapy must be tailored to address the individual meanings of every client.

Helping people revise rigid or outdated constructs that no longer serve the purposes for which they were devised is the goal of personal construct therapy. The spirit of this is captured by personal constructivism's notion of *constructive alternativism*, which holds that "all our present interpretations of the universe are subject to revision or replacement" (Kelly, 1955a, p. 15). Although we are not free to construe things any old way we like (after all, some constructions simply do not work well in navigating certain life circumstances), there are always countless alternatives to our current ways of making sense of things. Personal construct therapy maps people's constructs and encourages them to experiment with new ways of understanding the world.

For example, Mariska, a female, 32-year-old Black American, was divorced from her abusive ex-husband, Antonio. During their marriage, Antonio had been extremely controlling and manipulative. Mariska coped with this by pacifying Antonio—going along with his wishes, even at her own expense. When Antonio and Mariska divorced, Antonio insisted on custody of their 1-year-old daughter, Ada. Mariska sought therapy because she wanted shared custody of Ada. During therapy, Mariska successfully worked to become more assertive about her desires. However, a new issue emerged; now, rather than behaving complacently, Mariska found herself being extremely angry and combative with others—even in situations in which this seemed like overkill. Operating from a personal construct therapy perspective, I explored what the opposite pole of "complacency" was to Mariska. For her, not being complacent meant being "angry and combative." I suggested an alternative contrast to complacent: "persistent." Persistent people accept others' behavior (so they have no reason to be angry about it) yet persevere in pursuing what they want. Mariska found this suggestion helpful, and the following week reported that when Antonio had refused her request for a one-time change to their shared child custody schedule, she did not yell and curse at him. Instead, she persisted in assertively making her case, pursuing a compromise arrangement. This is an example of how personal construct therapy invitations to loosen and revise constructions can yield significant client change.

RADICAL CONSTRUCTIVISM

In a similar vein, *radical constructivism* views people's experiential realities as stemming from a "structure determined" combination of biological and psychological processes (Maturana & Varela, 1992). *Structure determinism* is the idea that the way an organism is built—its biological and psychological makeup—constrains and shapes how it can perceive, respond, and know. In other words, one's biological and psychological organization determine one's experience. For instance, a human being's olfactory system is different than that of a dog. Consequently, people and dogs differ in how they experience various odors—and even whether they smell them at all. Fido's snout registers fragrances that, for better or worse, a person's cannot. Smell is not simply an objective quality of the world; it is partly determined by the anatomy of one's nose. Similarly, although dogs can smell things that people cannot, people see colors that dogs cannot because the human visual system is arranged differently than a dog's. The human eye contains three rather than two types of cones, the photoreceptor cells in the retina that respond to color wavelengths (Rajalakshmi, 2023). Thus, the experiential reality of dogs and people is dictated by and emerges not as a perfect reproduction of the world but as something constructed by how their sensory and mental apparatuses respond when stimulated. The layout and design of organisms' perceptual and cognitive systems is what determines experiential reality.

According to structure determinism, people are *informationally closed systems* that are never directly in touch with the world itself. Rather, the world triggers meaning-making processes in the person, the results of which constitute knowledge (Glasersfeld, 1995; Maturana & Varela, 1992). Along these lines, radical constructivism assumes that people do not passively receive knowledge but, instead, actively build it up and that cognition serves an adaptive rather than a representative function—it evolved to help us survive, not to reproduce the world verbatim (Glasersfeld, 1995). For instance, human vision and bat sonar are different evolved mechanisms for navigating the world. Both are useful, but neither provides direct access to the world "as it is" (Raskin & Debany, 2018). Therapies stemming from radical constructivism presume "that the operations by means of which we assemble our experiential world can be explored, and that an awareness of this operating . . . can help us do it differently and, perhaps, better" (Glasersfeld, 1984, p. 18). The aim of such therapies is to disrupt the homeostatic status quo of people's structures to foster psychological reorganization.

Consider the case of Andrew, a 35-year-old man who sought therapy when he had difficulty ending the drastic diet that he had begun before attending a wedding. He began worrying that he had anorexia. The reason Andrew lost weight for the wedding was to compete with and outdo what he called the "cool kids" (now adults) from his high school who were also invited. Andrew had not been a cool kid in high school but had wanted to be—and suspected that his "pudginess" as a teenager had interfered with the cool kids liking him. Andrew sought to "beat" the cool kids at their own game, and his efforts paid off. At the wedding, he was as thin or thinner than any of the cool kids, many of whom had gained weight since high school. He had won! As Andrew explained it: "When I saw the cool kids at the wedding and they were heavier than I was, I knew I had finally beaten them." His therapist responded with a question: "So, you won a weight loss contest that your high school peers didn't know they were participating in?" This comment disrupted Andrew's understanding in a manner he had not anticipated. His "victory" suddenly seemed Pyrrhic. The diet, rather than a being victorious assertion of personal power, now seemed like a foolish and pointless act of possible self-harm. By the next session, Andrew reported that he had started eating and regaining weight. "Your question unsettled me," he told his therapist. "Once you asked it, I couldn't see things the same way." Consistent with a radical constructivist view, Andrew's psychological structure had been perturbed, resulting in rapid change because Andrew had to reorganize his understandings to reestablish equilibrium.

SOCIAL CONSTRUCTIONISM

Social constructionism offers a somewhat different (and complementary) view, maintaining that meaning is not as private and personal as personal constructivists and radical constructivists suggest (Gergen, 1995). Instead, meaning is something people create together through their ongoing relationships. How people talk, interact, and communally coordinate with one another through what social constructionists call "discourses" shapes their shared understandings (Burr, 2025; Gergen, 2015). That is, the *discourses* people develop—joint ways of talking and living—bring into being shared experiential realities. According to social constructionism, there are as many experiential realities as there are relationships (and the discourses that emerge from them). For example, "romantic love" seems like a universally true human experience, but social constructionism sees it as a discourse that offers "a framework to people within which they may understand their own experience and behaviour and that of others" (Burr, 2025, p. 84).

Thinking therapeutically, the discourses that constitute our lives and identities may not always be in our best interest. When embedded within the discourse of romantic love, one may purchase flowers and greeting cards for their betrothed to ensure that they remain enraptured. This might propagate capitalist economic arrangements that cause the person to feel inadequate and as if they are forever in search of additional purchases to guarantee the continuation of "true love." Social constructionist informed therapy challenges clients' internalized discourses about things, such as love, sex, gender, race, ethnicity, and religion. Because people are usually unaware of how internalized discourses operate and affect them, raising consciousness about these discourses is a key component of social constructionist therapy (McNamee et al., 2023). When people become cognizant of a discourse, it changes their relationship to it by making them aware of its status as a humanly invented way of understanding rather than a direct reflection of how things are.

For example, Dina, a 35-year-old lesbian woman, sought therapy for "low self-esteem." She viewed herself as a "nerd" and felt that her "nerdiness" prevented her from forming a meaningful romantic relationship. I asked her where the idea that she was a nerd originated, and she regaled me with stories about her high school experience and its social cliques—jocks, popular kids, and nerds among them. She had been labeled as a nerd in high school and come to experience and accept this as a key part of her identity. From a social constructionist standpoint, the discourse of "nerddom" predated Dina's arrival at high school; it constituted a social construction, one to which many people in her high school subscribed and—importantly—one that Dina, through her relationships in high school, had internalized.

Therapy consisted of raising Dina's awareness of the "nerd" discourse and challenging whether this was the only "lens" through which she could understand herself. As it had been many years since she had been in high school, Dina started to realize that the people she interacted with today did not necessarily see her as a nerd. In other words, the "nerd" discourse had little currency in her present relationships. Over the course of therapy, Dina deconstructed the discourse of "nerddom" and began experiencing herself quite differently. She was amazed to realize that a socially constructed classification of some people as "nerds" could have had such an enormous effect on her identity. Social constructions, although collectively made up, can be quite powerful when widely integrated into the social fabric, especially because their socially invented nature is typically overlooked. Social constructionist therapy works to remedy this by underscoring the social origins of our most cherished and taken-for-granted concepts.

INTEGRATED CONSTRUCTIVE PSYCHOLOGY

To simplify constructive theory for newcomers, key elements of personal constructivism, radical constructivism, and social constructionism can be combined into *four premises of an integrated constructive psychology* (Raskin, 2015; Raskin & Debany, 2018). These premises set the stage for thinking about how constructive theories can be used in psychotherapy.

Premise 1: People Are Informationally Closed Systems

According to the first premise, *"people are informationally closed systems, only in direct contact with their own processes"* (Raskin & Debany, 2018, p. 345). *Informational closure* is central to personal constructivism and radical constructivism. Both theories treat meaning as personal and private. They view people as in touch with nothing but their own internal experience. That is, human beings are only in contact with the world indirectly via their constructions of it. This means that the outside world we take for granted does not directly imprint itself on our senses. Sensory stimulation is the starting point rather than the end point. Instead of mirroring nature, it triggers meaning construction. Even when the outside world constrains meaning-making, it does not wholly determine it. A rock might strike me in the head, but the stars I see are a product of my visual system. The rock sets the system in motion, but the structure of the system—much more than the rock—determines what I ultimately experience. Likewise, when my boss upbraids me, the conclusions I draw about myself are not fully determined by the boss's tirade. From a constructive standpoint, my takeaway has as much to do with my self-perceptions, previous history with authority figures, the scuttlebutt of my coworkers, and so on. All of this is filtered through and constrained by my current psychological and biological structure.

Implications for Psychotherapy

The major implication of Premise 1 for psychotherapy is that therapeutic interventions—no matter how clever—do not directly instruct clients in how (or whether) to change. Clients respond to therapy based on their own unique structures. From personal and radical constructivist vantage points, no two clients respond to an intervention in precisely the same way. What works well with one client falls flat with the next.

When we view clients as informationally closed systems only in touch with their own processes, the goal becomes stimulating the system to reorganize it into a different configuration. Such prompting sets in motion new internalized meaning-making processes that generate novel experiences and outcomes. Constructive therapists are adept at stimulating mental reorganization, but precisely how understandings are psychologically restructured is determined by the parameters of each client's system. Remembering this guards against therapeutic hubris. Because therapists never directly "change" people in predictable ways, therapy cannot become an exact science with easy-to-apply formulas for success.

Case of Navin

Navin, a cisgender male college student, complained of loneliness yet stayed aloof from intimate relationships. Therapy focused on increasing his social engagement with others. Navin made progress but therapy ended prematurely when he moved away at the end of the academic year.

At our final session, as he was leaving my office for the last time, I stumbled over an unfortunately placed trash can by the door. With no therapeutic intention at all, I placed my hand on Navin's shoulder to steady myself and avoid losing my balance. A week later, I received a card from Navin in which he expressed deep appreciation for my final therapeutic act—touching his shoulder to convey what he construed as the grand theme of our work: the importance of human intimacy. Clearly, my clumsiness sparked an unexpected but favorable response in Navin. Had the same thing happened with another client, my touch likely would have triggered a totally different response (or, even more likely, no response at all!). From a radical constructivist perspective, when exposed to external events, people's psychological structures (and not events themselves) determine whether and how they respond.

Premise 2: People Are Active Meaning-Makers

The second premise builds on the first, holding that *"people are active meaning makers, drawing distinctions as they construct ways of understanding"* (Raskin & Debany, 2018, p. 346). Both personal constructivism and radical constructivism see people as actively devising psychological constructions. Personal constructivists view people as personal scientists who formulate hypotheses, which they then test and revise as they live their lives (Kelly, 1955a, 1955b). Similarly, radical constructivists maintain that each person builds an internal, subjective environment consisting of "repeatable objects" that are treated as existing independently in the external world (Glasersfeld, 1995).

Implications for Psychotherapy

Premise 2 implies that therapists should avoid seeing clients as passive victims of brain chemistry, environmental conditioning, or sociocultural determinants. Although these factors are highly relevant, people are not reducible to them. Constructive therapies treat clients as active meaning-makers struggling to create useful conceptualizations of their experiential worlds.

Case of Gina: Part 1

Gina, a middle-aged cisgender woman, worked as an administrative assistant in a small accounting firm. Her presenting concern was that she felt taken advantage of by others, including at work. Although her boss and fellow employees went to lunch each day, she remained behind in the office to answer calls. She believed she was expected to do this as part of her job and that taking a lunch break would anger her boss. It upset her that she never got to eat a proper lunch. Rather than conceptualizing Gina as possessing a pathologically "dependent" or "passive" personality, her therapist assumed that Gina's passivity reflected an active construal of the world informed by how she made sense of past events in her life. Gina reported previous experiences with aggressive men, some of whom had physically abused her when she failed to comply with their demands. Thus, she came to associate deference with safety.

In therapy, Gina was encouraged to actively develop a new hypothesis, namely that if she asked for a lunch break, her boss might grant it to her—a view that ran counter to her long-held belief that safety and assertiveness were incompatible. Gina tested this novel hypothesis by diplomatically and tentatively requesting a lunch break—and was pleasantly surprised when her boss (who had been unaware that Gina had been remaining behind while everyone else got lunch) did not respond angrily. Instead, the boss immediately scheduled a daily lunch break for Gina. By actively forming and testing a new hypothesis, Gina revised her meaning system and thus altered her circumstances. As this example attests, treating clients like active meaning-makers rather than sick patients has a great deal of generative potential.

Premise 3: People Are Social Beings

The third premise incorporates the social constructionist perspective, maintaining that *"people are social beings, using their intersubjective experiences to confirm the utility of their constructions"* (Raskin & Debany, 2018, p. 346). Although personal and radical constructivists tend to see subjective experience as personal and private, they recognize that we all must construe the construction processes of others—and in so doing, "we come to experience an *intersubjective reality*, which results when others respond to us in a manner that confirms our sense that they understand things as we do" (Raskin & Debany, 2018, p. 346). Social constructionism adds that personal construing is always informed by culturally shared discourses; construing never happens in a vacuum (Burr, 2025; Gergen, 2015). In other words, we are linguistic beings whose ways of understanding are constituted through language.

Although constructivist-oriented constructive theories stress people as informationally closed, social constructionist approaches highlight ways that people are "in touch" through how they talk and interact. People operate in language and share the world linguistically. Through language and social coordination, they come to experience a jointly shared, yet stable, reality.

Implications for Psychotherapy

Premise 3 expands conceptions of therapy to account more thoroughly for relationships (Procter & Winter, 2020). It also encourages awareness and critique of the broader social context:

> We may think of therapy as a venture in which the client and the therapist explore not only personal constructions, but also the discursive resources and practices that are culturally available. That way therapy incorporates a sort of discourse analysis in which both client and therapist participate as co-researchers. (Pavlović, 2011, p. 403)

Case of Gina: Part 2

In therapy, Gina began questioning socially shared discourses about masculine and feminine roles. Based on her prior experiences, she had always assumed that, as a woman, she needed to be deferent, polite, and "sweet" to successfully navigate the workplace. These social discourses about gender were incorporated into her personal construct system and had influenced her most important relationships—not just at work but also with her domineering and controlling boyfriend, Chad. However, as therapy progressed, Gina began to revise internalized views of gender roles. Doing so was not easy or linear; Gina often found it difficult to abandon long-held views she had internalized about her "proper" role as a woman. As Gina came to view many of her ideas about gender as socially constructed, she increasingly found herself less at the mercy of such ideas. This opened new behavioral vistas to her that had previously seemed unimaginable, including standing up to (and eventually breaking up with) Chad.

Premise 4: People Are Both Ontological and Epistemological Construers

The fourth premise holds that *"people engage in both ontological and epistemological modes of construing, alternating between them as necessary"* (Raskin & Debany, 2018, p. 346). *Ontological construing* presumes the existence of a world separate from one's understandings of it. When I slice a tomato with a knife, I construe both the tomato and knife as independently existing objects—just as I do pain and anger if I inadvertently cut my finger. Human beings construe ontologically most of the time, treating the distinctions they make about the world literally (as the territory, not the map). Doing so generally helps them function efficiently from moment to moment.

By contrast, *epistemological construing* occurs whenever people shift from treating their constructions as direct reflections of the world to viewing them as useful creations of their own nervous systems. When construing epistemologically, constructions can be called into question as people reorient their focus from understanding the world to understanding their understandings (Raskin & Debany, 2018). For example, scientists construe ontologically when they study the effects of gravity on falling objects, but they construe epistemologically when they scrutinize the very notion of "gravity" itself. Similarly, therapy clients construe ontologically when they consider how the Big Five personality traits affect their interpersonal relationships. However, they construe epistemologically when they question the utility of "personality" as a concept and treat it as an imperfect human notion devised to make better sense of experience. In other words, the goal of ontological construing is to grasp a presumed reality, whereas the goal of epistemological construing is to reflect on and reconsider the ontological constructions people ordinarily take for granted.

Implications for Psychotherapy

Being able to tack back and forth between ontological and epistemological modes of construing allows us great latitude in examining client constructs. Sometimes we treat these constructs as ontological reflections of the world. Other times we take a metaperspective and epistemologically call into question their origins, purpose, and utility.

Case of Toby

Toby, a transgender 35-year-old man, came to therapy complaining that his wife Kirsten was "mean and bossy." At times, Toby and his therapist construed ontologically, presupposing that Kirsten really was "mean and bossy." When they did this, they looked for strategies that Toby could use to cope with or alter his wife's behavior—a task he found somewhat beneficial. However, at other times, Toby and his therapist construed epistemologically, calling into question Toby's construal of Kirsten as "mean and bossy." They explored Toby's understanding of the terms "mean and bossy," including how he arrived at them and whether there were alternative meanings that he might consider. This led to Toby being asked to entertain the possibility that his wife's suggestions conveyed "care and concern" rather than "mean bossiness." As Toby did so, he began to experience Kirsten differently, which led him to respond to her in new ways that upended old patterns.

Like all of us, Toby alternated between ontological and epistemological modes of construing. He went from accepting his original construal of Kirsten as ontologically true to epistemologically questioning and revising it. Once Toby revised his construction of Kirsten, he quickly returned to ontological construing, treating his revised view as true. Toby is likely to keep regarding his new take on Kirsten as ontologically true until doing so fails to work—at which time further epistemological reflection may be required. As this example illustrates, people operate from an ontological place most of the time. Questioning whether one's experience reflects the "world as it is" only becomes necessary when taken-for-granted truths cease to function as expected.

WHICH THERAPIES CAN BE CONSIDERED CONSTRUCTIVE?

Constructive therapy is not a singular theory or method. The term "constructive therapies" is plural for a reason! Any therapy can be considered constructive if it both presumes people construct accounts of the world and it views therapy as an undertaking to help clients revise those accounts and experiment with new ways of living and understanding. The constructive therapies include personal construct therapy, coherence therapy, context-centered therapy, narrative therapy, narrative solutions therapy, and social constructionist therapy. The ideas in the next chapter draw from these different therapies, offering creative strategies for clinical practice.

4

The Therapy Process

Whatever exists can be reconstrued.
—George A. Kelly (1969e, p. 227)

The key to constructive therapies is helping clients to *reconstrue*— that is, to experience and make sense of events in novel ways that open fresh possibilities. To that end, constructive therapists use a variety of clinical strategies to encourage clients to test new ways of construing and behaving. This often involves raising clients' awareness of their roles in the meanings they rely on while simultaneously encouraging experimentation with alternative constructions. Such experimentation requires behaving differently to see where these shifts lead. Thus, despite constructive theory's reputation for being highly abstract (Neimeyer, 1997; Raskin et al., 2015), constructive therapy is anything but. It actively encourages clients to transform discussions held in the consulting room into concrete strategies that test novel ways of behaving and living in daily life.

https://doi.org/10.1037/0000468-004
Constructive Psychotherapies, by J. D. Raskin
Copyright © 2025 by the American Psychological Association. All rights reserved.

According to George Kelly, "The purpose of life is to be on with it" (Kelly, 1967, manuscript cover page). He explained:

> The key to therapy might be in getting the client to get on with a new way of life without waiting to acquire "Insight." After all, is that not the way man has been treating himself for thousands of years? Rarely does one know *where* he is going when he launches out into a new way of life, and even less often does he know what is wrong with the pathway he abandons. It is only in a semantically rationalized and elaborately psychologized society that one insists on knowing all the *whys* before seeking to experience the *whats*. (Kelly, 1966, p. 17)

This emphasis on concrete action sounds much like behavior therapy but differs from it by supplementing behaviorism's hard science "just the facts" objectivism with the subjective and idiographic aspects of humanistic and experiential approaches. According to psychotherapist Jay Efran, constructive therapy "preserves some aspects of the action-oriented and behavioral psychotherapies—the emphasis on problem solving and accountability—but it does not treat human problems simply as conditioned responses, skill deficits, or illnesses of the mind" (Efran et al., 1990, p. 21). Efran elaborated:

> Previously, therapists felt forced to choose between therapy as either an art *or* a science—and to construe themselves as idealistic humanists *or* hard-nosed realists. However, the new [constructive] epistemology makes it possible to synthesize useful elements from each of these positions and to better appreciate the connections between them. (Efran et al., 1990, p. 21)

ROLES OF THE CLIENT AND THERAPIST

In recent years, debate has arisen over whether to call those seeking mental health services *patients*, *clients*, *consumers*, *service users*, or even *survivors* (Casey, 2016; Costa et al., 2019; Priebe, 2021). This debate is interesting to constructive clinicians, who believe that language socially constitutes how we comprehend and experience the world. Constructive therapists tend to militate against medical model conceptions of their work (Efran et al., 2007; Kelly, 1955a; Leitner & Faidley, 2002; Raskin & Lewandowski, 2000). They dislike using biologized language to describe their craft, seeing what they do as rhetorical rather than medicinal: "Therapists have no salves to apply, no antibiotics to prescribe, and no surgical instruments to wield" (Efran et al., 2007, Accountability Redux section, para. 4). Instead, therapists are experts at discourse. They do not treat people; they talk to them. George Kelly understood this in the 1950s before it was popular to critique the medical model. He expressed skepticism about terms like "therapy" and "patient," remarking that reliance on this sort of medical terminology had negative consequences:

> The term "therapy" and its companion term "patient" carry many implications which we are reluctant to buy. Most of all, they carry the implication that the person served is reduced to an ultimate state of passivity and that his recovery depends upon his submitting *patiently* and unquestioningly to the manipulations of a clinician. (Kelly, 1955a, p. 186)

Terms like "patient," "client," and "therapist" remain popular—and, to avoid confusing readers, they are used throughout this book despite misgivings about them. However, thinking of the therapist as a "consultant" and the client as a "consultee" better reflects the therapeutic enterprise. The consulting room is just what its name suggests: a place for clients to consult with an expert adept at transforming taken-for-granted meanings and deconstructing linguistic quagmires.

Role of the Client

Consistent with a consulting model, constructive therapy sees clients as active meaning-makers, not passive victims of biology and history. Clients are stuck, not sick. Two metaphors nicely capture constructive therapy's active, nonpathologizing conception of the client's role.

As Scientist

The first metaphor is that of the *person as scientist*. This metaphor was advanced by George Kelly in his personal construct psychology. Kelly wondered why psychologists usually see themselves as actively forming hypotheses and predicting events but treat almost everyone else (including therapy clients) as passive and inert—"propelled by inexorable drives" (Kelly, 1955a, p. 5). In constructive therapy, clients are considered active meaning-generators. This puts them in the driver's seat. It means that they are forever in the process of making new predictions and revising old ones. In constructive therapy, clients are active participants expected to devise new hypotheses, test them outside the consulting room, and revise further predictions accordingly. In other words, "therapy sessions are thought of as laboratory sessions" in which clients and their therapists formulate hypotheses for clients to test during daily life, then refine and further implement (Viney, 1981, p. 272). Clients are treated not as sick patients but as personal scientists whose "behaviour is so clearly an experiment" (Kelly, 1970, p. 269).

Consider, for instance, Olive, a retired, 73-year-old, divorced woman who sought therapy because she felt overwhelmed by her ex-husband, who texted her multiple times a day. She felt obliged to respond, even when she did not wish to. Rather than treating her as a "deferent" or "dependent" personality, her therapist helped Olive develop an alternative hypothesis—namely, that she was not obliged to respond. When asked how she might test this, Olive said she could silence texts on her smartphone when not wanting to communicate with her ex. Acting as a personal scientist, she tested this hypothesis between sessions. To her delight, she returned the next week feeling much better. She had refined her construct system in view of her new experience.

As Discourse User

A second useful constructive metaphor is the *person as discourse user* (Burr, 2025), a social constructionist metaphor that incorporates social constraints more than the person as scientist does. It still sees people as active but acknowledges how socially shared discourses effectively limit possibilities. Although we are all privy to and influenced by many different discourses, we remain free to combine and reimagine them in a myriad of ways. For example, the discourse of "marriage" historically has defined marriage as between a man and a woman, whereas the discourse of "equality" holds that everyone has equal rights under the law. Mixing elements from both these discourses opened opportunities to use them in previously inconceivable ways—yielding a new discourse of "marriage equality." If the role of client is that of discourse user, then therapy becomes a place to clarify, refine, redefine, or resist the discourses that clients use yet take for granted.

Returning to the case of Olive, her deference was, in part, attributable to her internalization of traditional gender discourses, which presume that women should be pleasing and submissive. When therapy made these discourses explicit, Olive shifted from accepting them as unquestioned truths to resisting them. As Olive adopted more empowering discourses of femininity, her deferent behavior noticeably decreased.

Role of the Therapist

Constructive therapists regard with skepticism metaphors that portray psychotherapists as medical specialists who diagnose and treat illness. Instead, they view themselves as experts who use discourse and language to help clients invent and test new ways of making meaning. Thus, two helpful metaphors for the role of the constructive therapist are that of a research collaborator or philological consultant.

As Research Collaborator

If the client is considered a personal scientist, then the therapist's role becomes that of *research collaborator*. The therapist helps the client formulate the problem and generate testable hypotheses for addressing it. This encourages clients to construe events in new ways.

Consider, for example, Kanjira, a middle-aged woman who presented with feelings of despair following a recent divorce. As she and her therapist worked together, they identified loneliness as a key component of Kanjira's distress. The therapist asked Kanjira to brainstorm ideas for addressing loneliness. Because Kanjira was a voracious reader with a love for books, she and her therapist collaborated on a plan for her to join the local library committee, which was looking for new members. Kanjira did so and found the experience reduced her loneliness even though she sometimes found engaging with new people challenging. Her therapist continued to collaborate with Kanjira to help her refine and further test a variety of activities for addressing her loneliness while managing any accompanying social anxiety. As a research collaborator, the therapist's role was to treat Kanjira's loneliness as a problem rather than a pathology. The therapist engaged her as an active and agentic person facing life challenges and helped her to test and make sense of new ways of behaving.

As Philological Consultant

The constructive therapist's role can also be considered that of discursive expert—which, in keeping with the consultation model outlined earlier, makes the therapist a kind of *philological consultant* (Efran & Fauber, 2015). *Philology* is the study of language (Cambridge University Press & Assessment, n.d.). Because constructive therapists believe experiential reality is constituted by how people talk about things, the therapist's role is as decoder and clarifier of client utterances. The therapist "re-languages" the "explanatory fictions" in which clients get stuck.

Consider, for instance, Burt, a 45-year-old male client in the middle of a divorce. No longer living with his wife, Sheila, and 16-year-old son, Jeff, Burt believed he had "lost" his family—especially his relationship with Jeff. To Burt, "family" meant everyone living under one roof, regardless of how unpleasant it became. Family conflict extended beyond Burt and Sheila to Burt's relationship with Jeff. While living at home, Burt had always been the disciplinarian. In fact, Jeff became so angry with his father's heavy-handed disciplinary tactics that he began refusing to visit with him after Burt moved out of the family home.

Burt's therapist acknowledged and empathized with Burt's grief over the end of his marriage and his upset over his conflictual relationship with Jeff. However, the therapist challenged Burt's insistence that an "intact family" with Burt as chief disciplinarian was the only viable constellation. The therapist suggested that Burt try something new: Cede day-to-day discipline at home to Sheila and extend no-strings-attached dinner invitations to Jeff. Although Burt initially felt this meant abdicating his responsibilities as father and family man, he tried it—and quickly came to see that "family" and "father" need not be defined so narrowly. He could live outside the home and still be close to Jeff. He could also let Jeff's mother handle her share of disciplinary matters without ceasing to be an attentive dad. In acting as philological consultant, the therapist contested Burt's use of language, encouraging him to redefine family and fatherhood in broader and more flexible ways.

ROLE OF THE THERAPIST–CLIENT RELATIONSHIP

Conceiving of clients as personal scientists and therapists as philological consultants has implications for the therapist–client relationship. In the classic book *Persuasion and Healing*, Jerome Frank argued that psychotherapy consists of four elements: (a) a confiding relationship between a sufferer and a helper, (b) a healing setting in which sufferer and helper work together, (c) a rationale or myth that explains the sufferer's distress, and (d) rituals and procedures that helper and sufferer perform to remedy the sufferer's distress (Frank & Frank, 1991). Importantly, faith in the healing relationship may be more important than the rationales or remedies offered. Even the most suspect interventions can help when there is a socially shared belief in them: "Any ceremony believed in by both parties might do the trick" (Efran & Fauber, 2015, para. 8).

Although open to many rationales and remedies, constructive therapists nonetheless adhere to Frank's (Frank & Frank, 1991) conception of the "healing" relationship—even if their notion of "healing" is not in sync with a medical model of client distress; they use the term metaphorically rather than literally. Consistent with humanistic (and most other forms) of therapy, the confiding relationship and healing setting in constructive therapy offer clients Rogerian empathy, genuineness, and unconditional positive regard (Rogers, 1959). When clients feel heard, accepted, and loved, they are more open to change. But constructive therapy does more than just empathically listen to clients. Its central rationale is that distress results when people become locked into unhelpful ways of making sense of their lives. Although people's constructions may not replicate the world as it is, some prove more fruitful than others: "Some reconstructions may open fresh channels for a rich and productive life. Others may offer no alternative save suicide" (Kelly, 1969e, p. 228). The rituals and procedures of constructive therapy aim to open possibilities by perturbing the status quo and triggering novel ways of construing and behaving.

Thus, the therapist–client relationship in constructive therapy is collaborative, but its tone and tenor vary as do the strategies adopted. Constructive therapists draw from the full array of available techniques—directive, nondirective, interpersonal, cognitive, behavioral, humanistic, body-centered, mindfulness-based, family-centered, insight-oriented, and action-focused. Theirs is not a clinically driven approach that demands fealty to a delimited set of therapeutic strategies (Kelly, 1955a). Any ethical intervention that shakes up existing meanings while offering novel ways to construe events is fair game. The healing context and relationship take priority over loyalty to specific healing rituals. In this respect, constructive therapy is devoted to encouraging new meaning-making, not to privileging some techniques over others.

STRATEGIES/TECHNIQUES

What makes a strategy or technique constructive is not what the clinician says or does but whether it encourages clients to reimagine taken-for-granted meanings and actions. Thus, any strategy or technique engaged in with the goal of transforming client meaning-making can be considered constructive—including both those imported from other theoretical approaches and those invented on the spot. In other words, constructive therapies tend not to be strategy or technique driven. That being said, constructive therapists have developed a variety of unique therapy strategies and techniques that can be valuable additions to one's therapeutic toolkit. Some of the more common constructive strategies and techniques are discussed next.

Revising Personal Constructs

Like most constructive therapies, personal construct therapy is not technique driven. However, personal construct therapists have developed a variety of interventions and assessments that serve as helpful additions to the constructive therapy toolkit. These include adopting a credulous approach, mapping personal constructs, having clients enact fixed roles, working interpersonally using role relationships, and fostering coherence.

Adopting a Credulous Approach

The notion of a *credulous approach* derives from personal construct therapy. It is "a stance of openness and acceptance adopted by a clinician to understand how the client is presently experiencing the world" (Raskin & Morano, 2004, para. 1). Adopting the credulous approach means accepting what clients say, even when it does not fit with the presumed facts of the situation: "From a phenomenological point of view, the client—like the proverbial customer—is always right" (Kelly, 1955a, p. 322). The credulous approach communicates respect and curiosity about the client's experiential reality (Epting, 1984). In this regard, it is very much in keeping with the emphasis on empathy and positive regard found in person-centered humanistic therapy (Cain, 2010; Rogers, 1951, 1959). However, personal construct therapy is typically more directive than person-centered therapy. The personal construct therapist actively asks clients how they understand the world. Kelly gently poked fun at therapists who felt the only way to obtain information from clients was through indirect methods, such as nondirective listening, free association, dream analysis, or elaborate assessment techniques. His advice to therapists: "If you do not know what is wrong with a person, ask him; he may tell you" (Kelly, 1955a, pp. 322–323).

In addition to actively listening and working to comprehend client concerns, Exhibit 4.1 provides questions a therapist can use to credulously inquire about clients' presenting complaints. *Credulous listening*, in conjunction with questions like those in Exhibit 4.1, serves as "a kind of controlled yet compassionate phenomenological approach to understanding the client from the client's own point of view" (Epting, 1984, p. 9).

Consider, for instance, Elena, a 25-year-old Latina who presented with feelings of anxiety and depression. She felt she was "going crazy" but could not figure out why. I worked to credulously listen to and understand Elena's experience. She was in a long-term relationship with her live-in

> **Exhibit 4.1**
>
> **Seven Questions for the Elaboration of Client Complaints**
>
> 1. With what problems would you like help?
> 2. When were these problems first noticed?
> 3. Under what conditions did these problems first appear?
> 4. What corrective measures have been attempted?
> 5. What changes have come with treatment or the passing of time?
> 6. Under what conditions are the problems most noticeable?
> 7. Under what conditions are the problems least noticeable?

Note. Data from Kelly (1955b, p. 962).

boyfriend, Garth, whose angry outbursts were something Elena attributed to her failures as a supportive girlfriend. As part of credulously understanding Elena's experience, she provided the information in Table 4.1.

Through credulously elaborating Elena's complaint, it became clear to both of us that her anxiety and sadness were not a result of her failures as a girlfriend but her despair over Garth's behavior and her fear that she would have to suffer with it indefinitely. Although it took several months more of therapy and planning, elaborating Elena's problem proved enormously helpful. She eventually broke up with Garth, moved into her own apartment, and began developing new and more supportive relationships.

Importantly, using a credulous approach does not mean accepting all client utterances unquestioningly or as literal truths. However, it does mean that the therapist endeavors to comprehend client meanings rather than dismiss them as irrational falsehoods or reflections of underlying pathology. In taking a credulous stance, "it is very important that the counselor should not try to make everything fit logically, or conform immediately to the facts as externally perceived" (Epting, 1984, p. 9). In this respect, constructive therapy diverges from forms of cognitive behavior therapy (CBT) that focus on correcting clients' faulty thinking (Beck, 2019; Beck et al., 1979; Ellis & Joffe Ellis, 2019). From a constructive orientation, "irrational" beliefs are ones whose logic and meaning to the client the therapist has yet

Table 4.1
Elena's Responses to Seven Questions for the Elaboration of Client Complaints

Question	Response
1. With what problems would you like help?	"Feeling anxious and depressed; spending most days in bed."
2. When were these problems first noticed?	"Six months ago, which was 2 months after moving into my boyfriend Garth's apartment."
3. Under what conditions did these problems first appear?	"Whenever Garth and I had a big argument, usually one where he accused me of not being supportive of him—often when I made plans to do things without him or failed to be at the apartment when he arrived home from work."
4. What corrective measures have been attempted?	"I stopped seeing my friends without Garth and made sure to be there when he got home from work. It calmed Garth but did not improve my mood."
5. What changes have come with the treatment or the passing of time?	"As the months have gone by, it has become increasingly difficult to overcome my feelings of anxiety and depression."
6. Under what conditions are the problems most noticeable?	"When I'm at the apartment—either alone or with Garth."
7. Under what conditions are the problems least noticeable?	"When I call my mother or have opportunities to see my friends. Getting out of the apartment for any reason usually provides some relief."

Note. Data from Kelly (1955b, p. 962).

to grasp (Raskin, 2007). When a client expresses ideas that do not square with those held by the therapist, it is the therapist's responsibility to "lay out both versions side by side and not erase the client's version in order to replace it with the 'true' version" (Kelly, 1955a, p. 322). Thus, constructive therapists invite clients to consider alternative constructions or to entertain additional evidence without privileging their own account as the final, healthy, and correct one.

Consider, for example, the case of Melanie, a 40-year-old White woman who presented with obsessive thoughts about her late cat (Raskin, 2007). Melanie had long lived with her elderly and verbally abusive father. When the opportunity to move into an apartment of her own arose, she jumped at it. However, because the apartment did not allow pets, she brought her cat to an animal shelter, expecting it to be given a new home. Instead, the cat was put to sleep. Feeling distraught and responsible for the death of her cat, Melanie reneged on the apartment. She was convinced that her cat's death was the result of her selfish desire for independence and an apartment of her own away from her abusive father. Rather than directly confronting Melanie's beliefs as irrational, I offered an alternative construction for her to consider. After listening empathically to her latest lament about her selfishness, I remarked, "That's one way to look at it, but I have to admit that I don't see it that way" (Raskin, 2007, p. 61). This piqued Melanie's interest and led to the following exchange (Raskin, 2007, p. 61):

> "What do you mean?" she replied, cautious but curious.
>
> "Well," I said. "You pursued your own happiness for the first time in your life; unfortunately, things didn't work out and you concluded your cat's death meant you weren't supposed to be happy. From where I sit, that doesn't make sense."
>
> Melanie paused and then asked me, "You see it differently?"
>
> "Yes," I continued. "I think the part of you that wants to be happy finally got strong enough to put its own needs first, but then through some bad luck, things didn't turn out as planned. That was unfortunate, but it doesn't mean the part of you that feels you deserve to be happy was wrong."
>
> Melanie thought long and hard about this, laughed, and remarked, "You might be right."

In this exchange, I credulously listened to and accepted Melanie's construction of events. I did not treat her construal as irrational, wrong, or indicative of some underlying disorder. Yet neither did I accept Melanie's interpretation unquestioningly—as critics of constructive therapy insist is required based on the erroneous assumption that viewing accounts as constructed necessitates valuing them all equally (Ellis, 1997, 1998; Held, 1995, 1998; Mackay, 2011). Rather, I invited Melanie to entertain an alternative construction of events—one informed by my intimate understanding of how she made sense of things. Credulous understanding enhances the therapist's authority to challenge their clients. After all, "unless we can understand exactly why the loss of a pet was so devastating and what it was about a burglary that was so traumatic, neither good advice nor well-meaning interventions are likely to be helpful" (Butt & Parton, 2005, p. 804).

Mapping Personal Constructs

Assessment in personal construct therapy measures the personal constructs of clients. Rather than pigeonholing clients into nomothetic diagnostic categories, personal construct assessment unpacks idiographic meanings by identifying each individual client's unique bipolar construct dimensions. In so doing, therapist and client come to better understand how the client construes life and, based on this understanding, they can begin to experiment with alternative ways that the client might make sense of things instead.

Repertory Grid. One way that therapists can understand clients is by mapping their personal constructs. There are several ways to do this. Clinicians who wish to conduct a more structured assessment can administer the *repertory grid*, or "rep grid" (R. Brown & Chiesa, 1990; Fromm, 2004; Jankowicz, 2003; Procter & Winter, 2020). The rep grid is unique among appraisal measures in that it does not place clients into preordained categories in the *Diagnostic and Statistical Manual of Mental Disorders* (*DSM-5-TR*; American Psychiatric Association, 2022) or personality trait categories. Such classifications tell us more about how mental health professionals construe clients than how clients construe themselves. Instead, the rep grid identifies the unique personal constructs of each client—the bipolar abstractions people use to interpret events.

When administering a rep grid, the therapist typically provides the client with a list of *elements*. The focus of these elements can be anything the therapist thinks will help elicit the client's personal constructs. As a few examples, the elements can be people (e.g., mother, father, romantic partner, sibling, boss, favorite teacher, liked person, disliked person, admired person), aspects of the self (e.g., self now, ideal self, future self, how others see me), life events (e.g., birth, marriage, divorce, graduation), or even body parts—as has been done when eliciting constructs from clients diagnosed with eating disorders (e.g., legs, arms, face, fingers, waist;

Procter & Winter, 2020). Sets of three elements are presented to the client, who in each case is asked to identify one way in which two of the elements are the same and different (or opposite) from the third (R. Brown & Chiesa, 1990; Fromm, 2004; Jankowicz, 2003; Procter & Winter, 2020). The results of these comparisons constitute the client's personal constructs.

Consider, for example, Nicholas, a 21-year-old cisgender male college student. He identified his mother and favorite teacher as "kind" and saw his father as "tough," which he viewed as the opposite of kind. For Nicholas, "kind versus tough" was one of his personal constructs. After eliciting numerous personal constructs through successive presentation of "triads" (sets of three elements), this client was asked to rate on a scale (in some cases, a client is asked to rank order) each of the elements along all of the personal construct dimensions generated. Methods for having clients do this vary. See Suggested Readings and Resources at the end of the book for details. Table 4.2 presents the 7-point element ratings that Nicholas provided when evaluating the elements (in this case, people) used to obtain his personal constructs.

The rep grid not only allows clinician and client to identify the unique personal constructs each client uses to make sense of events but also to provide data on how clients apply their constructs to the group of elements used to elicit them. From a constructive perspective, the rep grid is a sophisticated and powerful *idiographic* (individualized) measure. Again, rather than forcing clients into preexisting diagnostic or trait categories, it tries to understand clients on their own terms.

Laddering. *Laddering* is a method to elicit and explore the implications of client constructs (Hinkle, 1965; Procter & Winter, 2020). It is a quick and easy technique for mapping and understanding client meanings. It is called laddering because it aims to metaphorically climb from lower level (*subordinate*) personal constructs to higher level (*superordinate*) ones that are more central and important to the client's worldview and identity (known as *core constructs*). In other words, personal constructs are organized in a hierarchy. Superordinate and core constructs rank higher than others; they carry more weight and greater implications. Laddering attempts to identify these higher level meaning dimensions. It begins by

Table 4.2
Nicholas's Repertory Grid Using a 7-Point Element Scale

					Element			
Construct	Mother	Father	Romantic partner	Sibling	Boss	Favorite teacher	Liked person	Disliked person	Admired person
"Kind versus tough"	1	7	2	5	7	3	2	7	5
"Happy versus annoyed"	3	6	3	4	6	2	1	6	3
"Anxious versus friendly"	2	4	6	6	4	5	7	2	4
"Arrogant versus quiet"	5	2	4	3	1	3	4	3	4
"Aggressive versus confident"	6	2	5	3	3	6	5	3	7
"Lets things go versus perfectionistic"	2	6	3	5	7	5	4	4	3
"Gets what they want versus cursed"	2	3	2	6	1	2	3	4	1

Note. Nicholas rated his personal constructs on a scale of 1 (*elements closest to the first pole of the construct*) to 7 (*elements closest to the second pole of the construct*).

eliciting a construct from the client, usually by asking the client to explain how two items are similar but different from a third. The items chosen need not be especially important to the client, and often it is helpful to pick three mundane objects about which the client does not have strong feelings. Once a construct is elicited, the client identifies the preferred pole and explains why that pole is favored. This explanation constitutes the preferred pole of a higher level construct. The client is then asked to provide the opposite of this new preferred pole, and the entire process is continuously repeated until the client is unable to generate additional constructs.

For example, consider Mike, a cisgender male client in his thirties who was asked to choose three makes of automobiles (he chose Ford, Chevrolet, and Toyota) and to explain how two are similar and different from the third. Mike said Ford and Chevrolet are "American" and Toyota is "foreign." Thus, "American versus foreign" was Mike's first construct. He was then asked which pole he preferred, and he indicated "American." His reason was that Americans are "strong," whereas foreigners are "weak." When asked why he preferred "strong" to "weak," Mike explained that being strong involves "being in charge" as opposed to "being at the mercy of others." Mike then described how "being in charge" is preferable because it ensures "staying safe," whereas "being at the mercy of others" implies "being victimized." The process continued until Mike could not generate further constructs. Notice how quickly Mike "laddered up" from a low-level construct ("American versus foreign") to constructs more core to how he comprehended himself, his relationships, and the world ("being at the mercy of others versus being in charge" and "staying safe versus being victimized"). Through laddering, Mike and his therapist came to better grasp Mike's presenting complaint: "I am socially isolated and perceived as intolerant and aggressive toward others who wish to impose their will on me." This complaint was clearly linked to the bipolar constructs Mike had devised to comprehend events, and helping Mike to revise these constructs became the focus of therapy.

Constructs at the bottom of a ladder tend to be concrete, whereas those higher up the ladder are more abstract. For instance, a married couple sought therapy to address recurrent arguments over trivial issues, and each began laddering from the construct "squeezes toothpaste tube from the middle versus squeezes tube from the end" (Procter & Winter, 2020). This highly concrete construct formed the bottom of their respective ladders, but the higher rungs for each of them were more abstract and informative. The next three rungs up the husband's ladder were "wasteful versus thrifty," "thoughtless versus conserves resources," and "exploits the planet versus respects the planet" (Procter & Winter, 2020). The wife's ladder yielded the higher level constructs "spontaneous versus inhibited," "authentic versus rule-bound," and "free versus repressed" (Procter & Winter, 2020). Laddering provided the therapist with a great deal of insight into how husband and wife differed in their meaning-making.

Other Techniques for Understanding Client Construing. Laddering is just one technique for understanding client constructs. Numerous other techniques have been developed, including *pyramiding* (Landfield, 1971), which, in contrast to laddering, "climbs down" the construct system from more central to less central constructs; the *ABC model* (Tschudi, 1977), which identifies how positive pole shifts on one construct have negative implications for pole shifts on other constructs; the *resistance to change grid* (Hinkle, 1965), which explores client preferences for maintaining rather than shifting from preferred construct poles; and the *implications grid* (Hinkle, 1965), which asks clients to rate the implications of changing poles on one of their constructs by checking off which of their other constructs they would also change poles on as a result. See Suggested Readings and Resources at the end of this volume for more on techniques for understanding client constructs; these techniques are perhaps most succinctly summarized by Procter and Winter (2020).

To briefly illustrate the utility of these techniques, consider how the implications grid helped Claire's therapist understand how moving Claire, a 44-year-old cisgender woman, from "angry" to "even-tempered" on one construct would also necessitate her shifting from "assertive" to "timid"—not something she or her therapist preferred. Thus, therapy with Claire must account for how changes in one area of her construct system ripple through and have repercussions for other ways that she construes herself and others.

Having Clients Enact Fixed Roles

Building on personal construct psychology's metaphor of the person as scientist, *fixed-role therapy* asks clients to play roles that diverge in important ways from how they presently construe themselves (Bonarius, 1970; Efran, 2024; Epting & Nazario, 1987; Kelly, 1955a, 1973). The goal is for them to "suddenly realize: 'If I *act* in a different way I can *be* different. I can be different from what I think I am. I can change'" (Bonarius, 1970, p. 213). The process usually begins by asking clients to write a self-characterization sketch of themselves in the third person from the perspective of a sympathetic person who knows them well. To help clients with this task, they are sometimes asked to write their self-characterizations as if written and sent by a close friend in the form of a letter to the client's therapist (Epting & Nazario, 1987).

Consider, for instance, Gigi, a 20-year-old transgender woman college student who drafted the following self-characterization sketch in which she described herself as "shy" and "socially avoidant":

> Gigi is a nice person, but other people often don't know this because she is painfully shy. She is so shy, in fact, that she will work hard to not talk to unfamiliar people, as doing so makes her nervous. It has come to a point where the other students at her college have probably given up on her, seeing her as a socially avoidant person who refuses to make eye contact or speak up either because she lacks confidence or doesn't care about other people. Gigi's social difficulties are made worse because she despises small talk. Even though she has a lot to offer, outside of occasional socializing with a few close friends, Gigi spends most of her time alone. As a result, she is lonely and depressed.

After clients share their self-characterizations, their therapists revise these sketches, altering them in ways that encourage experimenting with new forms of acting and living. The result is a *fixed-role sketch*, written (like the clients' original sketches) in the third person but given a different name than the client and altered in important ways. The fixed-role sketch should push the client to act in novel ways but not be so different from the client that implementing the role would be too difficult. Thus, Gigi's therapist provided her with the following fixed-role sketch of "Sammy," a private person who nonetheless engages comfortably with others when she wants to:

> Sammy is a nice person who sometimes feels anxious about socializing with others. However, Sammy doesn't let this stop her. When she encounters someone who is interesting to her, or when she feels lonely, she pushes herself to engage socially—or at least to not avoid others. Sometimes this means going either by herself or with a close friend to campus social events. Sammy cares about other people, even if the prospect of socializing is sometimes stressful to her. She also has enough self-confidence to see small talk and the occasional awkwardness of social gatherings as "necessary evils" for making and enjoying new friends. This perspective has generally worked for Sammy. Although she enjoys her alone time, Sammy has a reasonably active social life and only sporadically feels lonely.

After being provided a fixed-role sketch by their therapists, clients are asked to play their fixed-role characters in daily life, typically for 2 weeks. Continuing with the previous case, Gigi was asked to act like Sammy for a 2-week period. This included going to a campus party, something Gigi would never do. In her next therapy session, Gigi reported a remarkable experience: She attended a party like Sammy would, initially standing alone by the door. A few people came over and engaged her in discussion, offering her a drink and asking her to dance. To her great surprise, despite some lingering apprehension, Gigi found herself enjoying the party. Although she still did not consider herself a social butterfly, she continued periodically going to and having fun at parties, even after the fixed-role experiment ended. Sammy's more social comportment, initially foreign and frightening to Gigi, had been absorbed into Gigi's self-construction. This is the power of fixed roles. They reduce resistance to testing new behaviors.

Fixed-role therapy also proved helpful with Susan, a 24-year-old woman who presented for therapy with feelings of generalized anxiety, insecurity about her physical appearance, and shame over still being a virgin (Viney, 1981). Susan often felt others responded to her negatively.

Her therapist provided Susan with the fixed-role character of "Mary Jones," whose attributes were ones that Susan valued but was not embodying in her life. The fixed-role sketch read as follows:

> Mary Jones is a *friendly* young woman who is *open and frank* with the people she meets. She enjoys *giving* to these people and the feelings of *companionship* she has with them. She sees herself as *united* with her fellows, as *part of the world* with them.
>
> Mary is a *down-to-earth* kind of person, and most of the time she is *calm* and *relaxed*. She is able to be *patient* with the people she knows and is *not very critical* of them.
>
> Mary is also *searching* and *inquisitive* about her world. She can be *forceful* when the occasion demands it and *lively* too. Mary is the kind of person people like to know. (Viney, 1981, pp. 274–275)

Susan was asked to play Mary Jones between sessions. Initially she found this extremely difficult. "I couldn't possibly be like that!" she exclaimed (Viney, 1981, p. 275). Her therapist simply encouraged her to try out the role occasionally just to see what might happen. After some stops and starts, Susan eventually "tried the role briefly with a checkout woman in a supermarket and was surprised by how much more warm and friendly the checker became" (Viney, 1981, p. 275). A few weeks later, Susan tested the role again at two parties, where she did not know most of the attendees, as well as once at work with some colleagues: "What Susan learned from this experimenting was that if she thought and felt about herself differently, which she found she could do, people reacted to her differently" (Viney, 1981, p. 275). This insight helped her construe in new ways that better allowed her to anticipate and predict interpersonal engagements with others—thus, causing her less anxiety in such situations.

Working Interpersonally Using Role Relationships

Experiential personal construct therapy, developed by Larry Leitner, is a variant of personal construct therapy that places the interpersonal aspects of construing front and center (Faidley & Leitner, 1993; Leitner, 1988, 1995, 1999; Leitner & Faidley, 2002; Leitner & Thomas, 2003). It holds that "human meaning-making cannot be understood apart from the profound world of interpersonal relations" (Leitner & Thomas, 2003, p. 258). The most rewarding yet emotionally perilous thing one can do, according to experiential personal construct theory, is to grant another person access to the core ways one makes sense of self, others, and world. This type of closeness, in which two people construe each other's construction processes, is known as a *role relationship* (Kelly, 1955a). In such a relationship, "two persons are intimately interconnected through the mutual construing of the processes of the other" (Leitner & Thomas, 2003, p. 258).

Role relationships (which Leitner refers to as "ROLE relationships" to capture the deep and intimate way in which experiential personal construct psychotherapy conceptualizes roles) are critical to experiential personal construct therapy, which contends that sharing our deepest meaning-making processes with someone else is necessary because "people need profoundly intimate contact with others in order to live a life filled with richness and meaning" (Leitner & Thomas, 2003, p. 258). However, people often avoid this kind of intimacy because it is risky. Nobody wants their core ways of making sense of the world disconfirmed. Hence the irony: Role relationships are necessary to psychologically thrive, but they are also terrifying because they expose us to possible invalidation. In other words, the difficulty with role relationships is that they "may not only enrich but also may damage (even destroy) psychological life" (Leitner & Thomas, 2003, p. 258).

Role relationships are essential for mental well-being, but we often eschew them to prevent being hurt. The following questions can assess whether someone is retreating from role relationships:

> Is life rich, meaningful, filled with satisfaction and zest? Or is life basically empty, unemotional, meaningless? Can I say what I need to say to the others who are close to me or do I end up not being as open as I need to be? Do I truly feel like I understand the essence of the important others in my life? Do they believe that I really understand the central aspects of their being? Do I feel profoundly understood by these others? Do they believe they understand me in great depth? Trusting the client's experience around questions like these can be a profound indication of whether the client is excessively retreating from ROLE relationships. (Leitner & Thomas, 2003, p. 259)

The goal of experiential personal construct therapy is to help clients develop role relationships. Consequently, experiential personal construct therapy places the therapist–client-relationship front and center, using it as the central mechanism for change. In this regard, experiential personal construct therapy has much in common with interpersonal and object relations approaches that emphasize using the therapeutic relationship to provide clients with a "corrective emotional experience" (F. Alexander & French, 1946; Cashdan, 1988; Curtis & Hirsch, 2003; Levenson, 2017). Consistent with this, experiential personal construct therapy reimagines some relational psychodynamic concepts in constructive ways. It emphasizes the importance of constructs at a low level of awareness (Leitner, 1999). This echoes the psychodynamic notion of unconscious experience yet differs slightly because constructs at a low level of awareness are not wholly formed repressed memories to recover; rather, in keeping with the personal construct idea of *preverbal construing* (Kelly, 1955a), they are underdeveloped, unspoken, and tacit meanings to be verbalized, clarified, and reconsidered (Leitner, 1999). So, for example, only by talking with her therapist about her frustrations with dating does the client Melissa fully define, express, and bring into existence her preverbal construction that a relationship is "required" to "complete" her; once voiced, this construction is ripe for critical examination and potential revision.

Experiential personal construct therapy also appreciates the psychodynamic notion of *transference* but subtly redefines it in constructive terms as occurring when clients graft constructions of past relationships onto current relationships (Leitner & Thomas, 2003). For example, the core constructs of a client, Sally, paint people as threatening and untrustworthy. Transference occurs when she generalizes these constructs, developed in response to her abusive early relationships with her parents, to new relationships—including her relationship with her therapist (Raskin et al., 2005). Thus, Sally is extremely wary about sharing intimate life details in session and repeatedly worries that her therapist will break confidentiality.

To help clients like Sally, experiential construct therapists provide clients with a role relationship that is fundamentally different from those they have previously known. Thus, sessions often focus on here and now interactions in the consulting room. Like all constructive therapies, experiential personal construct therapy views each client as unique, and so the role relationships and in-session discussions about them must be tailored to each case. Use of structured manuals that script therapy is discouraged because manuals fail to account for the distinctiveness of each therapist–client relationship, inhibiting the establishment of transformative role relationships. Importantly, in calibrating role relationships, experiential personal construct therapists aim for *optimal therapeutic distance*, which requires being close enough to clients to intimately experience their feelings but distant enough to recognize their feelings as distinct and separate from one's own (Leitner, 1995).

To illustrate experiential personal construct therapy in action, let us revisit the earlier case of Melanie, the 40-year-old White woman experiencing obsessive thoughts about her late cat. During our sessions, Melanie often asked me for advice and opinions. I conceptualized this as a type of transference in which Melanie adopted a passive and deferent interpersonal style because she construed herself as meek and ineffective and others as dominant and knowledgeable. This way of interacting interfered with Melanie's ability to establish satisfying role relationships because she resisted saying what she needed to say. In session, I used a productive type of *countertransference* in which therapists monitor their responses to how clients construe and engage (Raskin et al., 2005). I shared my reactions with Melanie to help her explore how she meaningfully understood relationships. In an early session, when Melanie repeatedly asked me for advice about how to stop obsessing over her deceased cat, I responded as follows (Raskin, 2007, p. 57):

> "You ask me that a lot. . . . In fact, a lot of times when we talk, I feel like you want me to tell you what to do."
>
> "Well, shouldn't I? That's why I came here. I came here so you could tell me how to get over my problem." Melanie countered.
>
> "Fair enough," I replied. "But if I tell you what to do, will you do it?"

This question invited Melanie to consider the authoritative behavior she solicited from others, as well as her response when people accepted her invitation by telling her what to do. The exchange continued:

> Melanie smiled in response to my question about whether she would follow any advice I gave.
>
> "Yes," she said.
>
> "Even if you thought it was a bad idea?" I asked.
>
> "Yes," said Melanie. "I wouldn't want to be disrespectful. After all, you're the doctor."
>
> "Hmm. Do you ever do what other people besides me tell you, even if you think they are telling you bad ideas?"
>
> Melanie paused and thought for a brief period, before remarking "Yes, I do that with my mom all the time."
>
> As we discussed this issue, a theme emerged: Melanie looking to others for what to do, even when she has her own thoughts on the matter.
>
> "It seems that a lot of times you place other people's ideas about what to do and how to live above your own." I commented. "Are my thoughts about what you should do more important than yours?"
>
> "I don't know," she replied. "Maybe I think they are sometimes."
>
> (Raskin, 2007, p. 57)

Exchanges like this afforded an opportunity for me to discuss with Melanie similarities and differences between our relationship and the one she had with her mother, whose derision and judgment when Melanie did not "fall in line" influenced Melanie's construction that other people know more than she does and respond negatively unless she defers to them. Through sharing my reaction to Melanie's submissiveness in session, she acquired awareness of how she construed relationships. As therapy progressed, Melanie developed a more intimate role relationship with me in which she was increasingly less compliant and more willing to express her own opinions and desires. By the end of therapy, she had generalized these new interpersonal patterns of role relating to significant others in her life (Raskin, 2007).

Fostering Coherence

Coherence therapy is a constructive approach that combines the meaning-focus of personal construct therapy with neuroscience research on memory reconsolidation (Ecker, 2020; Ecker & Hulley, 1996, 2008). It emphasizes how coherent ways of understanding the world perpetuate client problems and symptoms. *Ways of understanding the world* are sometimes called "original learnings" because they frequently begin in childhood. They consist of powerful emotional learnings that inform cognitive schemas about how the world operates. These *emotional learnings* and *cognitive schemas* are basically ways of construing events. Coherence therapy is constructive in holding that "behind any current problem or symptom lies a compelling way of understanding how the world works that necessitates the presence of that problem or symptom" (Raskin & Bridges, 2024, p. 261). Each compelling way of understanding the world is personally constructed, but "once a construction of events is locked in, it becomes an unquestioned and largely unnoticed part of how the world is understood" (Raskin & Bridges, 2024, p. 261). Clients start treating it as a fundamental truth rather than as a constructed understanding. Yet, despite being implicit rather than explicit, original learnings are invented by those who use them. Although they often yield undesirable outcomes, they are conceptualized as limitations in meaning-making rather than as internal dysfunctions or pathology. Coherence therapy frees clients from these meanings by raising awareness of them in a way that transforms or dissolves them.

Consider, for example, Ethan, a male graduate student who presented in therapy with "procrastination" issues (Raskin & Bridges, 2024). His late submission of assignments was creating significant problems in his life, and he reported being "'just one out-of-ink print cartridge at the wrong time' away from failing out of graduate school" (Raskin & Bridges, 2024, p. 261). He had made many attempts to overcome procrastinating—including list-making, dividing work into chunks, making a schedule, and promising himself rewards for doing his work (Raskin & Bridges, 2024). However, none of these strategies had worked. Not only was his procrastinating the source of much personal anxiety, but it was also causing conflict with his husband, Mark. Despite Ethan's many apologies for his persistent dawdling, Mark's patience was growing thin (Raskin & Bridges, 2024).

In coherence therapy, symptoms are not viewed as signs of underlying pathology. Instead, they are seen as indispensable coping strategies that spring from unconscious meanings constructed by the client (Raskin & Bridges, 2024). Thus, his therapist set out to discover the unconscious meaning behind Ethan's procrastinating that made it compellingly necessary. The therapist asked Ethan to imagine what it might be like to complete his homework early. Although he initially indicated that this would feel wonderful, when invited to consider whether part of him would feel uncomfortable finishing his work ahead of time, Ethan paused and said yes (Raskin & Bridges, 2024). He indicated that if he finished early, his husband, Mark, would want to check his work for errors—and this would be painfully analogous to the intense criticism that Ethan had endured throughout his childhood and adolescence. Ethan did not want his relationship with Mark to become like those he was accustomed to in the past; his marriage to Mark had always been a relationship in which he felt unconditionally accepted. The mere prospect of introducing any kind of criticism into it—even constructive criticism—was unthinkable to him. Thus, procrastinating was a strategy for protecting his relationship with Mark and avoiding negative criticism like that he had endured in his youth. The unconscious meaning that emerged was that "corrections equal devastating criticism" (Raskin & Bridges, 2024, p. 262).

As he and his therapist processed this unconscious meaning in session, Ethan also became aware that sometimes he found corrections and criticism helpful—for instance, when learning guitar, playing soccer, and mastering calculus (Raskin & Bridges, 2024). Consequently, Ethan realized that equating corrections with criticism did not always hold true. This awareness corresponded to a marked decrease in his procrastinating.

> Because Ethan's constructed knowing that "correction always means criticism" and "correction can mean help" both felt true but could not be true at the same time, the more limiting of the two lost its hold on his life and allowed him more room to get his work done early. (Raskin & Bridges, 2024, p. 262)

In coherence therapy, when clients become aware of taken-for-granted unconscious meanings, symptoms often dissolve rapidly.

Shifting Contexts

Context-centered therapy is a constructive approach that emphasizes *contexts*, the sets of humanly devised assumptions that frame and organize experience (Efran & Soler-Baillo, 2008). Contexts, which are invented by people, consist of information that shapes and delimits what people can and cannot do. Contexts provide personally and socially constructed frameworks of meaning in which some things are possible, but others are not. In this respect, they are generative, bringing into existence domains in which certain explanations, actions, and forms of living become real and intelligible. Contexts allow certain domains of action while forbidding others. For instance, in the context of "chess," only certain things "go." The various pieces have names (e.g., pawn, rook, bishop) and ways they can be moved around the checkered square that forms the game board. Yet, only within the context of chess are these things true. When we shift contexts from chess to checkers, an alternative set of informational realities comes into existence. This is because contexts provide abstract borders within which certain types of action and ways of being are possible. As such, they both create and constrain. The analogy of a picture frame proves helpful. Typically overlooked, it is the boundary around a painting that allows us to identify "these particular blobs of paint as a work of art" (Efran & Soler-Baillo, 2008, p. 86).

Contexts are necessary for coherent living. They impose order on the jumble of information continuously flowing our way. They structure our experience, inform how we meaningfully understand events, and help us to establish goals (Efran & Sitrin, 2002; Efran & Soler-Baillo, 2008; Raskin & Efran, 2020). All human activity occurs within contexts. One cannot be a spouse outside the context of "marriage" or a "boss" outside the context of "the workplace." Likewise, it is impossible to be an "audience member" or "performer" unless operating within the context of "theater performance" or to be a "U.S. senator" independent of the context of the Constitution of the United States. These contexts provide the "space" or "structure" in which certain processes, explanations, and forms of action become possible, whereas others are prohibited or rendered incoherent. A non-kinged piece in checkers cannot move across the entire board in one move, but a queen in chess can. Similarly, an audience member cannot "divorce" disliked actors, but a disgruntled wife can do so to her husband. However, she cannot "impeach" him—unless she also happens to be a U.S. senator, and her husband is the U.S. president! Again, contexts create and constrain.

We all operate within a multitude of contexts, digitally moving from one to another in the blink of an eye. However, unlike picture frames, contexts are psychological and social inventions that do not exist in the physical world. This makes shifting among them something that occurs instantaneously. Reaching adulthood when the clock strikes midnight on one's 21st birthday, becoming a college graduate on crossing the stage at commencement, and attaining the status of spouse once the pastor pronounces you married exemplify the immediateness of contextual shifts. Speaking of marriage, context-centered therapist Jay Efran once noted,

> Finding a spouse can take years, but saying "I do" takes only an instant. Like all contextual transformations, the shift from "single" to "married" is *digital* rather than *analogic*—either/or rather than gradual. Although the processes they spawn unfold over time, contexts are instantaneously created and dissolved. (Efran & Soler-Baillo, 2008, p. 87)

The digital nature of contexts explains why, for example, Valeria, a 52-year-old female corporate executive, instantly transforms from boss to spouse when her wife, Anna, a 44-year-old female actor, picks her up at the office and why Anna switches from performer to friend on meeting an audience member for dinner after starring in the play. Sometimes contextual shifts proceed seamlessly, and other times, they cause difficulty. It can be hard to know how to act when we find our spouse present at a business meeting that we are running; the clash of contexts makes it difficult to determine which contextual rules to follow. Yet when contexts clash, we momentarily become aware of them. This is because contexts function as unspoken preverbal frameworks that shape meaning yet are easy to overlook. Contexts are potent and powerful but invisible to us when we are operating in them. We only become aware of them when they conflict or when we step outside them. It is not until my spouse interrupts my business meeting that I recognize the taken-for-granted unspoken frame that guides me at work. For a quick summary of the qualities of contexts, see Table 4.3.

Importantly, contexts evolve over time. Marriage used to be a context limited to one man and one woman, whereas now, same-gender marriages are "real," too, because the context of marriage has been extended. Similarly, Major League Baseball no longer allows all the infielders to play on the same side of the field; the humanly invented context of baseball has been revised to limit what happens within it. Although contexts do evolve, it can be a slow and difficult process because not only do contexts usually go unacknowledged, but they are also socially shared constructions—meaning that we usually cannot change them on our own.

Table 4.3
Characteristics and Examples of Contexts

Characteristics of contexts	Examples of contexts
■ Digital (not analogic)	■ Places (e.g., museums, theaters, schools, work)
■ Made of information (boundaries)	
■ Not fundamentally linguistic but can be encoded, accessed, and altered linguistically	■ People or relationships (e.g., marriage, business partner, friend)
■ Generative (bring into being some possibilities but not others)	■ Things (e.g., picture frames, chessboards)
	■ Roles (e.g., museum guard, waiter, teacher)
■ Precede (and contextualize) content and processes	■ Concepts (e.g., security, love, beauty)
■ Potent but easily overlooked	
■ Observable or noticeable only from the perspective of a larger context	
■ Can be widely shared across society or idiosyncratic to one or a small number of people	
■ Constrain and shape how aspects of the world "show up"	
■ Like all digital phenomena, are instantly transformable "outside of time"	

The only way for human beings to describe contexts is through language. How we talk about things matters. Language is not simply descriptive but constructive; it brings certain experiences into being while it simultaneously precludes others. However, the experiences one constructs are not to be confused with the world itself. The stories we tell establish the contexts that shape our experience. Hence, the configurations we impose bring lived realities into being. Marriage, gender, love, safety, and mental disorder are all contexts of meaning created through language. How we talk about things, alone and together, constructs contextual frames that we use to structure our lives—often for better, but sometimes for worse.

In context-centered therapy, mental distress is presumed to occur when people become trapped by contextual constraints. For example, operating from a context that places "security" front and center, a client assumes they must endure the drudgery of their nine-to-five job; it is only when the client shifts to a context emphasizing "satisfaction" that quitting their day job to pursue an acting career emerges as an option. Becoming contextually ensnared like this is easy because, despite their importance, the contexts in which we operate often remain largely invisible to us. We typically treat language as descriptive rather than constructive, so the contexts we build tend to be implicit rather than explicit. Therefore, when people fail to recognize the context-based presumptions that bring certain lived realities into being, they treat them as literal truths and get stuck. It is because contexts often go unnoticed—serving as unquestioned backdrops yielding immutable impressions—that people become locked into troublesome and distressing patterns.

Context-centered therapy focuses on shifting clients from their usual contexts to novel or unfamiliar ones that open new vistas of possibility. This is accomplished through simply fostering awareness. Taken-for-granted but troublesome contextual assumptions are made explicit, and then clients are invited to do nothing more than notice when they are operating from them. This works because it is impossible to observe a context from within that context. Thus, the straightforward act of awareness necessitates contextual shifts.

Consider, for example, Suniko, a 30-year-old cisgender woman who presented with generalized anxiety. She worried about everything. She dreaded giving presentations at work, feared driving her car because she might get into an accident, and fretted about (and avoided) socializing with others because she might say or do something "dumb." She was convinced there was something fundamentally wrong with her but sought therapy based on a slim hope that it might help. I told Suniko that anxiety was a normal and expected human experience and gave her a simple assignment: to simply observe and note (rather than try to stop) her anxiety reactions between sessions. This task has similarities to currently popular "mindfulness" interventions (Hayes et al., 2004; Langer, 1989; Teasdale, 2004). Consistent with the mindful emphasis on inquisitive openness, the constructive rationale was to invite a contextual shift, moving Suniko from a stance of judgment and condemnation to curiosity and acceptance. To her great surprise, she returned the next session to report far fewer instances of anxiety ("It really didn't happen that much this week"), and when anxiety did rear its head, it was far less intense. From a context-centered therapy perspective, the simple act of awareness works because to observe a problem-generating context, one must shift to another, larger context—and this usually results in significantly different ways of interpreting and experiencing the world.

Like personal construct therapy, context-centered therapy is not technique focused. It supports all interventions that encourage contextual shifts. Next, I discuss three context-centered strategies that constructive therapists often use: (a) orthogonal interaction, (b) encouraging awareness of mind and self, and (c) depersonalizing life.

Orthogonal Interaction

Orthogonal interaction occurs when someone responds to us differently than we are used to, eliciting novel reactions (Efran & Sitrin, 2002). Consider, for example, Kiran, a 19-year-old male client who has kept threatening to drop out of college and may have become accustomed to friends and relatives trying to talk him out of it. He likely has expected more of the same from his new therapist. However, by engaging orthogonally, his therapist has increased the chances of generating change. One way the therapist could engage orthogonally is by agreeing with Kiran that dropping out of school might be best. This response is orthogonal because it is unexpected. Consequently, it is more likely to elicit something different from Kiran than were the therapist to merely echo the sentiments he is used to hearing. The therapist's unanticipated response might result in Kiran finally feeling free to really drop out of school. Or, it might result in Kiran becoming less enamored with dropping out; absent the usual pushback against his threats to quit school, Kiran—to his own surprise— might even find himself inclined to complete his degree.

As this example illustrates, by forcing the client to respond to something unforeseen, orthogonality potentially provokes new thoughts, feelings, and behaviors—keys to effective therapy. It encourages contextual shifts and the reorganization of how one meaningfully construes and experiences events. In radical constructivist terms, orthogonality disrupts the homeostasis of people as structure-determined systems, forcing rearrangement into a new configuration. This is a technical way of saying that sometimes we have experiences that initiate immediate and irreversible changes over which we have no control. These can be minor (e.g., being told that cherry soda tastes like cough syrup, leading to it no longer tasting good) or major (e.g., reading a book that transforms one's understanding of the world or, more problematically, going through a traumatic event that fundamentally alters how one experiences self and world). Orthogonal interactions can yield positive or negative changes. Context-centered therapists try to generate the positive changes. However, even though non-constructive therapists do not invoke orthogonality as an explanatory concept, all effective therapy can be viewed as requiring orthogonal engagement with clients:

> The principle of orthogonality takes advantage of the fact that all of us are capable of a much larger range of behaviors than we typically enact. Because the therapist is outside the client's ordinary milieu, he or she can trigger responses that in other settings are unavailable, underused, suppressed, or prohibited. (Efran & Sitrin, 2002, p. 139)

Take, for example, Cody, a 22-year-old Asian American male client who presented with feelings of jealousy about his girlfriend remaining friends with her past boyfriends. Cody was accustomed to people telling him he needed to "get over" his jealousy to fix his "possessive personality."

With that end in mind, his previous therapist had encouraged Cody to alter the "irrational thoughts" behind his jealousy. Unfortunately, the more Cody tried to do this, the worse his jealousy became. He understood that his jealousy was not rational, yet he continued to experience it. By the time he sought therapy with me, Cody felt utterly defeated but decided to give therapy another chance to "cure" his jealousy.

I interacted orthogonally with Cody by telling him that jealousy was not a defect in his personality but an evolutionarily baked-in (albeit unpleasant) response. I suggested that he accept it and the irrational thoughts that accompany it. This was not what Cody was expecting at all! Startled by my take on the issue, he could not fall back on his usual responses: angry outbursts followed by apologies and a toxic mix of anxiety, guilt, and self-pathologizing. Instead, he laughed and relaxed. Then, he began to imagine what a relief it would be if he let himself off the hook when jealousy arose. To his surprise and pleasure, by the time he returned for a second session, Cody's jealousy had diminished substantially and, when it did make an appearance, he found himself far less bothered by it. My orthogonal interaction with him—in which I responded in a manner different from what he anticipated—forced Cody to engage his jealousy in a fresh way.

Understanding the power of orthogonality offers a way forward whenever therapists feel uncertain about how to proceed with clients. That is, "when therapists are unsure about what to do, they ought at least to do something different from what other people in the client's life are already doing" (Efran & Sitrin, 2002, p. 139). Expanding on this, the principle of orthogonality reflects the context-centered view of therapy as

> a social influence process, more akin to education and politics than to science and medicine. In a sense, the therapist ferments small revolutions in the consulting room by engaging clients in orthogonal interaction. These encounters change the client's purview, allowing hidden assumptions about life to be aired. (Efran & Sitrin, 2002, p. 140)

Orthogonality offers a highly potent therapeutic tool, one that can be seen in most of the interventions outlined in this volume.

Encouraging Awareness of Mind and Self

"Mind" and "self" are two contexts that can be especially helpful in developing clinical conceptualizations (Efran & Soler-Baillo, 2008; Smothermon, 1980). Context-centered therapists define these terms in unique ways. They do not treat mind and self as fixed and essential personality traits. They instead view them as goggles that, when looked through, shape how we experience events (Raskin & Bridges, 2024). As we move through life, we all vacillate between the contexts of mind and self.

The context of *mind* very narrowly frames the world in strictly defensive and self-protective terms (Efran & Soler-Baillo, 2008; Raskin, 2023; Raskin & Bridges, 2024; Raskin & Efran, 2020, 2021; Smothermon, 1980). It focuses exclusively on safety and survival. This is because, as far as the mind is concerned, self-protection and maintaining control reign supreme. To the mind, there is nothing worse than being wrong, which it experiences as akin to "losing." The mind dreads the vulnerability it associates with losing or being wrong; it insists on always "winning" and "being right." In other words, "the mind keeps itself safe by trying to dominate and control others and by avoiding all risk. It never moves beyond its 'protect and defend' orientation; while it serves an evolutionary purpose, happiness is not on its radar" (Raskin & Bridges, 2024, p. 262). For example, when Tammy operates from mind, she opts to remain isolated and alone rather than risk rejection by engaging with other people. She might yearn for more social connection, but so long as she views the world from the self-protective context of mind, safety will continue to trump happiness.

The context of *self* is broader than that of mind. Instead of dwelling on safety and self-protection, its focus is on empathy, connection, and affinity with others (Efran & Soler-Baillo, 2008; Raskin, 2023; Raskin & Bridges, 2024; Raskin & Efran, 2020, 2021; Smothermon, 1980). When we act from self, we adopt a stance of generosity, understanding, compassion, and gratitude. We accept others and meet them where they are, being careful not to shame them or make them feel "wrong" or "one down." We encourage them to be "mindfully" self-aware of when they are operating from the context of mind, and how this can interfere with their well-being. Such awareness requires moving from mind to self because one can only observe the mind from outside it—in this case, from the broader context of self. Importantly, context-centered therapists do not try to stop the mind because, from a structure-determined radical constructivist perspective, the mind is not something one can directly control. Counterintuitively, the only way to loosen the grip of mind is to observe and accept it—something we saw previously in the case of Suniko overcoming her generalized anxiety. When therapists encourage acceptance of the mind's defensive postures, they orthogonally interact with clients who are accustomed to others treating their mind-based behaviors as signs of disorder that must be discontinued.

Consider, for instance, Cecil, a male, 76-year-old, retired advertising executive who presented in therapy with debilitating anxiety over potentially moving to a luxury retirement community for seniors. He had lived with his wife Patty in the same house for 50 years, and although they loved their two-story, five-bedroom home, they increasingly felt overwhelmed by having to maintain it. Still, Cecil was terrified at the prospect of upending his secure and familiar existence. Consequently, to Patty's chagrin, whenever she raised the idea of moving, Cecil negated it and experienced a panoply of mind-based responses in which he envisioned all sorts of disastrous scenarios. He feared moving away from his familiar neighborhood and agonized that downsizing to a smaller living space would force him to throw away items he "couldn't live without." He also worried incessantly about whether he and Patty could afford the retirement community, and he convinced himself that—even if they did move—they would never find doctors as good as those they were leaving behind. When all else failed in responding to Patty's increasingly desperate entreaties that he consider the move, he resorted to the panicked argument that moving might be the "wrong decision."

Rather than getting into a win–lose battle over the wisdom of the move, Cecil's therapist explained the difference between mind and self and commented that our minds always become activated when seriously pondering major life changes; after all, the sole focus of the mind is to keep us safe, not happy. The therapist further predicted that Cecil's mind would continue to "do its thing" whenever exploring the move but that observing the mind in action might prove beneficial. As Cecil began attending to his mind-based responses, he found they became less intense and more infrequent. He also found himself increasingly open to and less threatened by the idea of moving. After a visit and tour of the retirement community, he was surprised by unexpected feelings of excitement; he had begun shifting to a self-based stance of curiosity, openness, and adventure. Always "at the ready" to fight perceived threats, Cecil's mind did not completely stop "doing its thing," but he gradually found himself able to step beyond the mind into a broader, self-based orientation. Six months after Cecil and Patty pulled the trigger on their move, he told his therapist that it was the smartest decision they had made in years. He still found himself occasionally plagued by the mind's doubts and worries, but he no longer felt paralyzed by these experiences.

Therapists opting to incorporate mind and self into therapy can speak with clients about common mind–self contrasts, which are outlined in Table 4.4. As clients start applying these terms to their everyday lives, they often find themselves less beleaguered by their minds.

Depersonalizing Life

Because people's responses are structure-determined by how their systems are configured, every individual's behavior is always about them rather than us. In other words, life is not personal—even though it often feels like it is. As examples, when a friend does not return Debbie's phone calls, she concludes that she is unlikable and not important enough to be called back. When Bill's boss fails to praise his most recent earnings report, Bill infers that his work must be so dubious that his boss refuses to acknowledge it. Debbie and Bill incorrectly interpret others' behavior as about them instead of attributing it to others' temperaments and experiences. Perhaps Debbie's friend has a track record of not returning calls, or maybe her friend is experiencing a debilitating depression. Likewise, Bill's boss might be stingy with praise, or they could be handling an office crisis and not yet be able to read Bill's report. Even when someone's behavior is pointedly directed at us—as when Victor goes out of his way to bully and abuse his colleague Sandra—it still is not personal. It is hurtful and

Table 4.4
Mind Versus Self in Context-Centered Therapy

Mind	Self
Survival: Makes others wrong, blames, judges, operates from a self-protective/defensive stance	*Living*: Seeks connectedness and interrelatedness; nonpossessive, unselfish, open, generous, accepting, loving
Blame: Finds fault, makes others wrong	*(True) responsibility*: Acknowledges own role in how one experiences circumstances
Insufficiency: Perceives survival resources (both physical and psychological) as lacking; leads to selfishness	*Sufficiency*: Acts from conviction that the world is bountiful and there is enough for all; materially and psychologically generous
At effect: Views oneself as victim of circumstances (bad luck, perniciousness of others, events beyond one's control)	*At cause*: Takes charge and makes choices to care for oneself and serve others, even if unable to alter material circumstances
Avoidance: Steers clear of what seems frightening or risky; avoids facing psychologically or physically threatening issues	*Mastery*: Faces threats and works to cope with or overcome them

Note. From Table 1 in "Using Context-Centered and Person-Centered Therapies to Unite a Divided Nation," by J. D. Raskin, 2023, *The Humanistic Psychologist*, 51(1), p. 4 (https://doi.org/10.1037/hum0000276). Copyright 2022 by the American Psychological Association.

unfortunate but not personal. Something about Sandra sets Victor off, but this only informs us about Victor's system and what it responds to. It tells us very little about Sandra and how she operates.

The idea that life is not personal is counterintuitive and difficult to bear in mind, especially during taxing interactions with others. After all, it seems like their behavior is about us. Why else would they be acting toward us as they do? Because we observe other people's behavior and then experience our own reactions to it, we often deduce a link between them—especially when we are stressed and operating from the defensive and self-protective context of the mind. What we are not privy to, but which are equally if not more important, are the processes in others that guide their responses; people do indeed react to us, but each in their own structure-determined way. Given how easily people miss this, it is common for them to initially express skepticism when confronted with the idea that life is not personal. Nonetheless, with many clients, teaching them to not take others personally can be a powerful intervention.

For instance, consider Brynn, a 20-year-old cisgender female college student who sought therapy for bullying. She had been on her university's soccer team, but after sharing concerns about how the team was being run, she became the object of ridicule by her teammates. Initially, they verbally abused her but later progressed to ghosting her: They stopped returning her texts, speaking to her during team meals, or acknowledging her presence on bus trips to games. This caused Brynn a great deal of distress, and she eventually quit the team in despair despite her love of soccer.

When she began therapy with me, Brynn was convinced that her "distasteful and opinionated personality" was primarily to blame for her teammates' rejection. I wondered aloud whether she was adding insult to injury by taking the dreadful behavior of her soccer teammates personally. She found this hard to fathom, noting that it must have been her outspoken disposition that led them to mistreat her; had it not been, they would have chosen someone else to target. Because she struggled to grasp the notion that life is not personal, in an early session, I asked her to name two foods: one she liked (she said fish) and one she disliked (liver). I then asked her to think of someone whose tastes diverged from hers: someone who disliked fish but liked liver. She thought of her mom. I then inquired whether this difference in taste preference told us about liver and fish or about her and her mom. Brynn suddenly recognized that it told us about her and her mom. "Exactly," I replied. "Your dislike of liver is not personal to liver; it is about how your particular taste buds (compared with those of your mom) respond to it." This led to a lengthy discussion about how other people might respond to Brynn differently (perhaps more positively) than her soccer teammates—even though that, too, like her and her mom's responses to liver and fish, would not be personal.

Brynn decided to test this hypothesis by trying out for the lacrosse team. She made the team and was surprised to find herself warmly welcomed by her new teammates. Unlike her experience on the soccer team, her lacrosse teammates liked her very much—especially her "outspoken" way of raising issues, which they felt helped address those issues to the benefit of the team. By the time Brynn finished therapy after 3 months, she had learned that even when other people responded to her in ways she found disappointing, it was not personal. Invoking another food analogy, she concluded that "I will never be everyone's cup of tea, and I'm fine with that."

Even in the most intense family scenarios, the notion of life as not personal can be powerfully effective. For example, Julio, a 35-year-old married man, came to therapy because of feelings of inadequacy. Throughout his childhood, Julio's father had been physically abusive toward him. Like many abused children, Julio both felt responsible for what happened to him and guilty over his periodic feelings of rage toward his father, who, by this time, was elderly and unwell. As Julio's therapist, I asked him to imagine an alternate universe in which everything was the same except that Julio's father had a different son instead of Julio.

"In this alternate universe, would your father have treated this other son similar to how he treated you?" I inquired.

"Yes. Absolutely," Julio replied immediately.

"Well," I said. "Then what you experienced was awful and unfortunate but not personal. It wasn't about you. It was about your dad."

This insight stopped Julio in his tracks. He had never entertained the notion that his father's behavior might be independent of him. He had always assumed that he was the cause of his father's anger. Julio found himself resonating with the idea that what he lived through, although terrible, had never been personal. When Julio returned for his next session, he reported that his anger toward his father had not made an appearance since our previous meeting and that he had been feeling less negative about himself as well. Helping clients to depersonalize situations can be a powerful tool in the therapist's arsenal.

Revising Stories Together

From a social constructionist standpoint, "therapy can be described as a process of meaning making, where clients and therapists jointly create understandings about people and their dilemmas, as well as what can be done about those dilemmas" (McNamee et al., 2023, p. 26). Central to therapies informed by social constructionism is the idea that meaning-making is not done in isolation. It is always done in collaboration with others and influenced by broader cultural themes (Burr, 2025; Gergen, 2015). Socially constructed "discourses" constitute shared stories that bring certain lived realities into being. They are best understood as collective understandings and ways of life that are developed and maintained in conjunction with others and as socially invented rather than discovered (Burr, 2025; Gergen, 1994, 2015).

People erroneously assume that because social constructionists contend that ways of understanding are "made up," change occurs easily by just discarding earlier accounts in favor of new ones. However, it is not that easy. Once people create and share social constructions, these constructions take on a life of their own and can be quite resistant to change. Returning to an earlier example, "marriage" is a social construction; people invented it to understand and structure relationships. However, over time, the discourse of marriage became taken for granted as a true reflection of nature rather than a socially invented conception. Its origin as a jointly made-up scheme for understanding the world grew obscure as it came to influence how people defined themselves and others. This clarifies why expanding the scope of marriage to same-sex relationships was prolonged and difficult: The original way people came to mutually define marriage became reified, inhibiting new possibilities.

Consequently, the idea of marriage as "between a man and a woman" was beyond question to many people. Suggesting otherwise was to "deny reality." This illustrates how once others settle on socially constructed discourses, these discourses prove extremely hard to escape or overturn. As another example, the teenage boy labeled a "wimp" by his peers may find it incredibly challenging to move beyond the socially constructed ways that others view him. He may even find it difficult not to define himself in these same terms! Although the discourse of "masculinity" from which "wimpiness" emerges is a human creation, it takes on enormous power once shared widely and internalized by people. The therapy strategies discussed next—externalizing the problem, minding the gap, identifying nominal fallacies, and identifying microsocial and macrosocial processes—help clients recognize and resist overlooked relational discourses that contribute to their mental distress.

Externalizing the Problem

Narrative therapy contends that the stories people construct—alone and in concert with one another—are responsible for the psychological quagmires in which they find themselves (Monk et al., 1997; Monk & Zamani, 2019; White & Epston, 1990). We often mistakenly assume that our *narratives*, the socioculturally influenced stories we tell, reflect the world as it is. That is, we forget that our stories are merely stories and not reality itself. Because they are stories, they can be revised and retold. *Narrative therapy*, an approach focused on helping clients retell constraining stories, is one of the more popular constructive approaches. Consequently, it has garnered an exclusive volume elsewhere in the American Psychological Association Psychotherapy Series, where it is reviewed in detail (Madigan, 2025). Here, I provide a succinct overview of the approach, highlighting the constructive elements of one of its main techniques: externalizing the problem.

Narrative therapy challenges individualistic and medicalized conceptions, arguing that they yield pathologizing stories (White & Epston, 1990). Pathologized stories lock clients into unhelpful identities that portray them as broken and sick.

Consider, for instance, Agatha, a 19-year-old female therapy client whose self-narrative depicted her as "shy" and "anxious." Whenever the prospect of engaging others arose, this unhelpful story got in her way by attributing her problem to immutable personal characteristics. "How can I talk to others? I am shy and suffer from crippling anxiety!" she exclaimed to her therapist. The goal of narrative therapy is to help clients like Agatha revise their *problem-saturated stories*, stories that fuse them together with their problems. Externalizing the problem disentangles people and problems and, in doing so, nicely illustrates the narrative approach.

The premise of *externalizing the problem* is straightforward and simple. Rather than seeing problems as disorders inside of people (conditions they "have"), externalizing invites clients to view and talk about their problems as separate and distinct from (i.e., "external to") themselves (Tomm, 1989; White & Epston, 1990). In other words, the client is not the problem; the problem is the problem. Externalizing can initially seem odd to clients, especially if they are accustomed to telling themselves problem-saturated stories. Returning to the case of Agatha, a therapist using externalizing would ask Agatha to talk about her shyness as if it were a discrete entity, one that often gets the best of her.

Once the problem is distinguished as separate from Agatha, she and her therapist can begin *mapping the influence of the problem*. Mapping entails asking questions, such as: "What role does the problem have in your life?" "In what ways does the problem act like it's your friend when it's not?" "When are you most vulnerable to the influence of the problem?" "Who in your life would be least surprised at your ability to stand up to the problem?" (Raskin & Bridges, 2024). Questions like these help clients to identify times when they are most vulnerable to the problem. They also help pinpoint *exceptions*—instances when the problem had less of an influence over them. Distinguishing occasions when the problem exerts less influence allows clients to recognize *sparkling moments* (also called *unique outcomes*) during which they have effectively avoided falling prey to the problem. Highlighting these moments brings small victories into focus and serves as the starting point for telling a new story about the problem, one in which the client can overcome or outfox it (Madigan, 2025; Monk et al., 1997; Raskin & Bridges, 2024).

Agatha might be encouraged by a narrative therapist to externalize "shyness." Rather than thinking about shyness as a fixed and innate quality, she would be instructed to talk about it as something separate from her that often gets the best of her. She would give it a name, such as "The Big Shy," and be encouraged to treat is as an independent entity rather than an internal personality trait. This would allow for a discussion of how this externalized being gets the best of Agatha. Her therapist would ask questions, such as:

- When does "The Big Shy" have the greatest influence over you?
- What strategies does "The Big Shy" use to get you to go along with its wishes?
- Can you recall times in your life when you resisted the influence of "The Big Shy" or when "The Big Shy" was less of a force in your life?

The goal of questions like these would be to help Agatha identify when she is most vulnerable to "The Big Shy" and when she successfully outmaneuvers it. As Agatha increasingly recognizes that "The Big Shy" exerts greater sway over her in some circumstances than it does in others (e.g., when she goes to social gatherings alone rather than when she goes with a friend), she could begin identifying concrete strategies for effectively resisting it.

Raising awareness of exceptions to the problem's influence helps clients discern problem-fighting strategies that work (and which they already use!). Externalizing upends dominant internalizing, problem-saturated narratives (e.g., Agatha is, at core, a shy and anxious person who is incapable of social engagement). It replaces them with new narratives that distinguish person from problem (e.g., Agatha can thwart shyness by inviting friends along on what would otherwise be daunting social outings). By externalizing shyness, Agatha comes to embrace a new and more productive story, one in which shyness is an adversary that she can resist rather than consider an internal flaw. Externalizing is a creative way to help clients reconstrue themselves and their circumstances.

Minding the Gap

Narrative solutions therapy integrates narrative therapy with elements of personal construct therapy, solution-focused therapy, strategic therapy, and person-centered therapy (Eron & Lund, 1993, 1996, 2002). It holds that people experience mental distress when their behavior and other people's responses to it are inconsistent with their *preferred view*—the ways they prefer to see themselves and prefer others to see them. The idea of preferred view has similarities to person-centered therapy's notion of the self (Rogers, 1959), except that rather than being an innate aspect of the person, it is posited as a constructed way of seeing oneself (Eron & Lund, 1996). Thus, in a narrative solutions approach, a person's preferred view is never written in stone:

> Let us be clear that we do not see "preferred view" as a "thing" that people "have" and cannot get rid of. Rather, we are talking about a host of possible views or preferences that suit people, that fit with who they wish to be. For example, "I'm clever," "I'm a good mother,"

"I'm a good thinker," and "I'm sensitive and caring," may all represent preferred attributions of self. (Eron & Lund, 2002, p. 73)

Consider, for instance, Horatio, a man in his late twenties who wishes to see himself as "courageous." This is his preferred view. However, he encounters psychological upset when a gap occurs between his preferred view of himself as "courageous" (for rock climbing without safety gear) and his family's view of him as "foolhardy" (for taking excessive risks). Horatio also experiences distress when he fails to live up to his own preferred view by behaving in a "cowardly" manner (when he fails to stand up to his tyrannical boss). Narrative solutions therapy alleviates mental distress by reducing or eliminating gaps between preferred view and behavior as well as preferred view and how others view us.

Consider the case of the Ryan family (Mr. and Mrs. Ryan) and their two adolescent children: daughter, Jean, and son, John, who presented in therapy with intense family conflict—mainly between Mr. Ryan and Jean (Eron & Lund, 2002). In their first session, the family recalled a typical argument, which involved Mr. Ryan arriving home from work and criticizing Jean for eating on the sofa instead of doing her homework. Jean, in turn, dismissed her father's concern ("Lighten up dad. Are you stressed out from work or what?"; Eron & Lund, 2002, p. 68). Mr. Ryan then called Jean "lazy," and Jean "responded with an obscenity" (Eron & Lund, 2002, p. 68). Mrs. Ryan tried to keep the peace by asking Mr. Ryan to calm down, but this only made matters worse. Recurring conflicts like this were the reason the Ryans sought therapy.

The Ryan family's therapist, Tom Lund, spoke separately to Jean and her parents. When speaking to Jean, he began to understand her preferred view. Jean wanted others to perceive her as smart and effective. She recalled times from her childhood when her dad saw her this way—specifically, when he was impressed by how quickly she had mastered skiing and golf: "He taught me. I did good. . . . He would tease his friends about how I was going to beat them all before I left junior high school" (Eron & Lund, 2002, p. 78). However, despite her strong high school grades, Jean no longer felt that her father viewed her as smart: "All he does is question how I get such good grades when I can't remember to do things that he asks me at home. . . . I can't stand him anymore" (Eron & Lund, 2002, p. 78). There was a gap between Jean's preferred view and her sense of how her dad regarded her, and this prevented Jean from being able to behave according to it:

> The more convinced Jean became that her father thought her to be stupid, incompetent, and unworthy of his respect, the more she wore her defiance like a badge, concealing her preference for closeness and masking her sadness with sarcasm and anger. (Eron & Lund, 2002, p. 79)

Similarly, there was a gap between Mr. Ryan's preferred view (as a father who—unlike his own father—remained close to his daughter and involved in her life as she grew up) and how he thought Jean saw him (as someone she no longer loved or needed). In this light, Mr. Ryan's increasingly desperate attempts to be "involved" in Jean's life by providing "input" on what she was doing "wrong" became understandable, even though these efforts were terribly ineffective.

When told of Jean's positive skiing and golf memories, Mr. Ryan agreed things had been better between them in the past. Asked why, Mr. Ryan replied that Jean used to be "interested in what I had to say" (Eron & Lund, 2002, p. 79). The path forward involved helping the Ryans to appreciate one another's preferred views. Once Jean understood that her father did not see her as "stupid" and merely wished to be involved in her life, she no longer felt compelled to resist and dismiss his input. Likewise, Mr. Ryan was able to shift his behavior once he grasped that Jean, rather than wishing to be free of him, was hungry to be close to him while also wanting him to see her as smart and capable. In narrative solutions therapy, reducing the gap is key to clinical success.

Identifying Nominal Fallacies

If we view the categories people use to understand themselves as socially constructed, then treating these categories too reverently (as objective discoveries rather than communal inventions) risks imprisoning people within classificatory schemes of their own making. This results in *nominal fallacies* wherein we mistake the names we use to describe ourselves for explanations of behavior. This can quickly bog down therapy:

> Not only do clients come in with a host of beliefs, images from the past, fixed attitudes, and false causal assumptions, therapists often add their own explanatory fictions to the mix, introducing hazardous abstractions such as ego-strength, frustration tolerance, insecure attachment, automatic thoughts, negative schemas, unprocessed memories, and so on. Even common clinical terms such as *anxiety* and *depression* can be more of a hindrance than a help. (Efran & Fauber, 2015, para. 54)

When therapists and clients take the explanatory fictions they use too literally—"terms like *anxiety, self-esteem*, and *ego strength*" (Efran & Fauber, 2015, para. 55)—they risk closing off avenues of exploration by overlooking the specific meanings clients use and the circumstances they face. "Curing anxiety," "increasing self-esteem," and "boosting ego strength" are abstractions; it is difficult to measure when they have been achieved. By contrast, "speaking up at work," "asking someone on a date," and "resisting peer pressure from friends to smoke" are concrete goals unencumbered by vague professional jargon. Thus, the constructive therapist works with clients to describe problems in ordinary language. Doing so encourages the development of clear goals and concrete solutions.

Consider, for instance, Tamara, a 35-year-old female client with a bipolar diagnosis who often went on expensive shopping sprees. She attributed her shopping sprees to "being bipolar." This provided a comforting yet circular account that explained little. Tamara went on shopping sprees because she was bipolar. How did she know she was bipolar? Because she went on shopping sprees! Accepting this explanation limited therapy to working around the margins, helping Tamara manage her bipolar disorder. However, more extensive change required moving beyond the bipolar diagnosis to explain Tamara's behavior.

Working constructively, Tamara's therapist asked what was happening in her life before her last shopping jaunt. Tamara recalled an upsetting argument with her spouse. The ensuing discussion in therapy about this argument generated an alternative hypothesis in which Tamara shopped to feel better after distressing events. Asked to track this going forward,

Tamara recollected other upsetting occurrences that coincided with the urge to shop: conflicts at work, difficult phone calls with her mother, and feeling socially isolated from her friends. From there, she and her therapist entertained ideas for how Tamara might handle future instances of distress; instead of going shopping, she could discuss the situation with those involved. At her next session, Tamara reported having talked through a disagreement that occurred with her spouse. They resolved the issue, and Tamara did not go on a shopping spree. This marked the beginning of a sea change in Tamara's behavior. The more she confronted rather than avoided interpersonal conflicts, the less she felt inclined to shop.

Recognizing nominal fallacies is a key strategy in the constructive therapist's tool kit. When clients alter the language that they use to describe themselves and their behavior, downplaying essentialized labels that offer illusory explanations, new possibilities appear.

Consider the case of Elliott, a 22-year-old cisgender man whose involuntary outpatient treatment following a psychotic break included social skill-building sessions during which he practiced interviewing for jobs. Elliott became quite adept at mock interviews, so much so that his therapist felt Elliott was ready to pursue real job interviews. Elliott disagreed: "I can't go on real interviews!" he exclaimed. "I'm a schizophrenic!" Therapy involved helping Elliott change the language he used to describe himself. Even though Elliott did not reject his diagnosis entirely, he came to see it as a poor way to explain what he could or could not achieve. Social constructionist perspectives on therapy discourage overly individualized explanations relying on nominal fallacies that tightly link behavior to fixed internal attributes.

Attending to Microsocial and Macrosocial Processes

From a social constructionist perspective, therapy—like life—is socially constructed. Everything about it is "made up" (e.g., its notions of health and pathology, its theoretical models, its interventions)—literally brought into being through how we talk and interact together. Social construction occurs on both microsocial and macrosocial levels. *Microsocial processes* refer to specific interactions among people (McNamee et al., 2023), so, using an example, when Corwin seeks therapy from Dr. Grossi, the two of them coordinate when they will meet, where sessions will take place, the forms of payment that are acceptable, and the kinds of conversations they will have. Other therapists and clients may do these things differently; the specifics of "how therapy is done" vary widely. Thus, microsocial processes are the local, on-the-ground forms of coordination between people (McNamee et al., 2023).

By contrast, *macrosocial processes* are the broader discourses that frame and contextualize microsocial processes (McNamee et al., 2023). Corwin and Dr. Grossi may idiosyncratically coordinate the specifics of their therapy, but this occurs within a larger set of social discourses and practices that they cannot escape or avoid. For all the uniqueness of their therapy dyad, Corwin and Dr. Grossi have internalized (and likely take for granted) socially constructed discourses pertaining to "mental health," "therapy," and "capitalism." Importantly, microsocial and macrosocial discourses mutually influence one another. For example, microsocial processes between Sigmund Freud and his early patients were initially completely unique to them, such as meeting in 50-minute intervals to discuss the patient's difficulties (Will, 2018). However, widespread adoption of this practice contributed to the macrosocial discourse in which the "50-minute hour" is regarded as an essential feature in the practice of what we now call "therapy." Macrosocial discourses about therapy affect the microsocial processes of therapists and patients everywhere, but they are also affected and altered by the spread of new microsocial discourses—unique ways of construing that develop between two (or among a few) people, which bring into being new discourses along with corresponding patterns of interpersonal engagement and self-understanding (McNamee et al., 2023). Perhaps this is why psychodynamic, humanistic, and CBT forms of therapy have both influenced and been influenced by one another.

BRIEF VERSUS LONG-TERM WORK

Those who favor brief therapy emphasize its efficiency and cost-effectiveness (Lynch et al., 2021; Shapiro et al., 2003). By contrast, those who prefer long-term therapy express a preference for "depth"—deep and meaningful change that occurs over time (Michaels, 2020). Constructive therapists appreciate both perspectives but do not typically draw a firm distinction between brief and long-term work. Because they view change as digital (i.e., an instantaneous response to interventions), they believe it happens quickly—a stance consistent with brief therapy. Yet, they also recognize that people must integrate the implications of digital changes. In some cases, this occurs rapidly, but in other cases, it takes time—a view consistent with long-term therapy. Recognizing that each person works through change at their own pace, constructive therapists see no significant difference in the processes or procedures underlying brief versus long-term work—and do not privilege one over the other. They work with their clients for as long as it takes to help.

For example, consider Sasha, a 28-year-old cisgender female client who presented with generalized anxiety. She felt anxious about many things, including speaking in meetings at work and socializing with friends and family. In each of these situations, Sasha worried about being evaluated negatively by others. Her therapist introduced the idea of life not being personal, and once Sasha grasped the idea, it was like a light bulb had gone off. The change was instantaneous! She returned the next session and reported that she had experienced very little anxiety in the intervening week. Thus, therapy ended up being quite brief. After three sessions, Sasha thanked the therapist and indicated further sessions were unnecessary. She had gotten what she needed. This example illustrates how constructive therapy can be quite brief; when change is digital, its immediate effects are often speedily assimilated into people's lives.

But this is not always so. Even though the digital nature of change means it occurs in a heartbeat, not all therapy winds up being brief. Sometimes clients need time to integrate change, even when they have previously "gotten" it.

Consider, for instance, Alex, a transgender man who first came to therapy in his early twenties. His primary complaint was obsessive thinking; he regularly became overwhelmed by feelings of inadequacy about which he endlessly ruminated. Therapy focused on Alex's observing and accepting these thoughts as they occurred along with teaching Alex about mind and self. As a result, Alex quickly shifted to experiencing rumination as his mind's attempt to keep him safe. This produced a sharp decrease in how much he ruminated. Nonetheless, Alex continued to encounter times—usually when under stress—during which his ruminating returned with a vengeance.

Alex continued in weekly therapy for 2 years, finding it helpful to keep talking about his rumination and to hear his therapist repeat lessons about it articulated in earlier sessions—namely, that it reflected Alex's mind at work. These therapeutic conversations allowed Alex, over an extended period, to integrate his new awareness and understanding. Even after Alex's symptoms decreased sufficiently for him to stop attending therapy on a weekly basis, he periodically contacted his therapist for "booster" sessions. Change may be digital, but many clients find making sense of it and incorporating it into their lives come more slowly. In such cases, longer-term therapy is called for. Therapeutic duration varies, but constructive principles of change remain constant.

OBSTACLES IN USING THIS APPROACH

Constructive therapy challenges many of therapy's "sacred cows." This can create obstacles for therapists curious about the approach, although it can also attract clinicians who like to "think outside the box." Several examples of these "obstacles" are discussed next.

De-Emphasis of the Medical Model

Being a constructive therapist requires a subtle shift in professional identity—from disorder expert to discursive expert (Efran & Fauber, 2015; Raskin & Lewandowski, 2000). Instead of seeing themselves as master diagnosticians who objectively identify mental disorders, constructive therapists view themselves as philological consultants whose expertise is in talking with people in novel ways that elicit new responses (Efran, 2020; Efran & Fauber, 2015). This contradicts the medical model that remains prominent in training and practice (Wampold & Imel, 2015). It may be hard for some clinicians to cease viewing therapy through medical goggles—a challenge exacerbated because many of them work in systems requiring medical-style diagnoses for third-party reimbursement. Nevertheless, constructive therapists generally regard diagnostic systems, such as the *DSM-5-TR* (American Psychiatric Association, 2022), as imperfect inventions created by clinicians (Raskin & Lewandowski, 2000). They sometimes use diagnostic labels for practical purposes (e.g., to quickly convey basic information or collect insurance reimbursements). However, they urge caution when doing so because, from a constructive perspective, diagnostic language typically reveals more about the meaning-making of the professionals doing the diagnosing than the clients being diagnosed. If a therapist's goal is to understand how clients make sense of the world, then professional diagnostic terminology is of limited utility (Kelly, 1958/1969c; Raskin & Lewandowski, 2000).

Further, because constructive therapists conceptualize the clinician as a creative conversationalist rather than a diagnostic specialist, they are loath to rely on manualized interventions (Bohart et al., 1998). Manuals provide structure and direction to therapists—especially insecure new trainees looking for a script to guide them. However, constructive therapy adopts an idiographic stance, meaning that it sees each client (and therefore each therapy case) as unique. Thus, effective therapy demands not just empirically supported treatments but also artistry and creativity (Efran & Fauber, 1995; Leitner & Faidley, 1999; Raskin, 1999). Therapists seeking the certainty and security that more structured and manualized approaches provide may be reluctant to adopt a less scripted constructive stance.

The Past Is Not Privileged

Constructive therapy ascribes no special importance to past events. Thus, it disavows the common belief that therapy must focus on the past. Instead, constructive therapy emphasizes the "now." After all, "there is only now—the past and the future are language inventions" (Efran, 2022, p. 9). People invoke the past to explain the present and predict the future. The past becomes yet another explanatory fiction that merely explains how we currently construe events. However, despite the stories we tell ourselves about the past's influence, our history need not dictate our future. For instance, Aidan may not have asked anyone on a date last year, last month, or yesterday, but he is free to do so this afternoon. Likewise, Adrianna's recent failure to seek new jobs following several prior professional disappointments may affect her optimism about landing something, yet it does not prevent her from applying for a newly advertised position at work.

Constructively speaking, behavior is an experiment (Kelly, 1966, 1970). Therefore, one is always able to try something new. Unfortunately, many therapists retain allegiance to a backward-looking approach that focuses on "explaining" client problems. This can prove an obstacle to their adopting a constructive perspective. Nonetheless, therapists are invited to consider whether the past is all it is cracked up to be.

Therapy Length and Session Duration Questioned

Most constructive therapists are still agnostic in the enduring long-term versus short-term therapy feud; they decide the length of therapy case by case. Building on this, constructive therapists show no special allegiance to the 50-minute hour. Just as they figure out the number of sessions based on the time necessary to address client concerns, they also may decide the duration of individual sessions by how long it takes to deal with the issues at hand.

Constructive therapist Jay Efran remarked that "the notion that therapy sessions should begin and end at a set time was an invention of clinicians, not clients" (Raskin & Efran, 2020, p. 5). He questions this tradition, arguing that "although some issues can be dealt with in just a few minutes, others require more than an hour to resolve" (Raskin & Efran, 2020, p. 5). Therapists may appreciate this sentiment in theory, but it can prove impractical in modern practice—especially for those who accept health insurance. Although some therapists charge by the session, insurance companies pay by the hour. Admittedly, although constructive therapists appreciate the wisdom of not being confined by the clock, implementing this in practice remains an obstacle for most of them.

No Standing Appointment Times or "Termination"

Along similar lines, constructive therapy questions whether having "standing appointment times" for clients is helpful. From a constructive vantage point, it is a bad idea to maintain regular weekly meetings with clients regardless of the status of the therapeutic work. Doing so encourages therapy as a way of life rather than as a means of getting people "unstuck" and moving forward. Although standing appointment times sustain a reliable income for therapists, it is unclear how this helps clients. People do not keep in continuous touch with their dentists; they call when they need a teeth cleaning or have a toothache. Too often, therapists and clients keep meeting regularly simply out of habit, under the assumption that clients—even when "better"—require ongoing therapy lest they backslide into pathology. This results in therapeutic aimlessness, exemplified by recurring yet fruitless sessions of little urgency or accomplishment. No other profession works this way. I do not call the doctor to let them know I am feeling well, nor do I contact the plumber to tell them the sink is working. I do keep the plumber's phone number handy, however—and a similar model is part of a constructive approach to therapy. Client appointments are scheduled as needed, sessions typically occur in chunks, and clients are never "terminated" (i.e., we finish with them "forever").

Consider, for example, Albert, a male client in his forties who came to therapy after being laid off from his job. We met regularly for a while, during which we unpacked and processed Albert's evolving constructions about his career. We "depersonalized" his firing, helped Albert grieve the loss, and developed plans for Albert to reenter the work world. After 3 months, Albert had a new job and was feeling much better. After several sessions of his regaling me with his latest on-the-job successes, we decided that regular appointments were no longer necessary. However, I did not "terminate" the therapy relationship. Rather, I told Albert to call in the future should issues arise that he wished to discuss. A few months later, when Albert received a mediocre performance review from his new employer, we had a "booster" session to reinforce the themes of our prior work. A year after that, Albert contacted me when he was unhappy with his new job. We met for four or five sessions, during which he decided to go back on the job market.

The language of "termination" tells us more about therapists' ideas concerning saying goodbye to their clients than it does about clients' desire to keep seeing us. Constructive therapy is problem focused: Therapist and clinician define the problem to address and then work to reframe its meaning in ways that yield change. Given that new problems arise in all clients' lives, open-ended standing appointments and once-and-for-all termination are unnecessary. This runs counter to how many therapists conduct their practice.

Changing Contexts Is Harder Than It Looks

Approaching things from a different context or meaning framework than the client is necessary for effective constructive practice but can be difficult to do. Embracing the same contextual assumptions as the client prevents the clinician from provoking transformational change. Yet, moving beyond the client's contextual milieu can be quite difficult; it requires both identifying and then stepping outside the client's constructed assumptions. This is easier when therapist and client do not share the same allegiances (Efran & Fauber, 2015). Sharing a worldview can be comforting, but it risks therapists inadvertently reinforcing rather than upending client preconceptions.

Consider, for example, Karen, a heterosexual, 40-something, divorced woman. I had worked with her during her divorce, but now—a year or so afterward—she sought therapy again following the breakup of her first postdivorce relationship. Brian, the man she had been dating, was charming and fun to spend time with, but a committed relationship was not something he wanted. He therefore would go for prolonged periods without contacting Karen or responding to her texts. She found herself feeling angry and hurt because she wished for a more serious relationship. She wanted a clean break from Brian and asked me to help her "get over" him.

We agreed that the best way to do this was for Karen to stop texting and calling Brian as well as to pursue dates with other men. Karen did these things but to no avail. She was unable to stop obsessing about Brian and the wonderful relationship they could have if only he would commit to it. What prevented me from being an effective therapist in this case was that I had become ensnared in the very same contextual assumptions as Karen: She wanted to stop thinking about Brian, and I took that on as a goal. In doing so, I accepted her contextual frame that having feelings about Brian was bad and something to eliminate. In a more productive approach, I would have encouraged Karen to indulge and even act on her feelings toward Brian. Had she done so, Brian would have come around or continued his reticent behavior toward Karen. Either way, these new experiences with Brian were more likely to shift Karen in a new direction than trying to deny her feelings for him.

By treating Karen's ongoing interest in Brian as she did—as something problematic to eradicate—I failed to move beyond the contextual frame she brought to the situation. Approaching things from a different frame in which her feelings for him were okay, to be accepted, and to be abided by would have had a better chance of shifting the status quo. As in this case, all therapists sometime become trapped within their clients' contextual assumptions. It is a professional hazard that can be quite difficult to avoid. Thus, the need to identify and challenge contextual assumptions can prove an obstacle to working as a constructive therapist. Being an effective therapist means remaining on the lookout for assumptions that interfere with engaging clients orthogonally.

5

Evaluation

Science is not just a collection of laws, a catalogue of unrelated facts. It is a creation of the human mind, with its freely invented ideas and concepts.
—Albert Einstein and Leopold Infeld (1938, p. 310)

There are two big challenges in evaluating constructive therapies. First, constructive therapists have a long track record of studying the efficacy of their approach but, like their psychodynamic and humanistic peers, they value a diversity of research methods and do not always privilege randomized controlled trials (RCTs; Bohart et al., 1998). Consequently, constructive therapies are sometimes unfairly accused of lacking empirical support. Second, constructive therapies have a reputation for being highly abstract and theoretical—a problem constructive therapists have inadvertently contributed to by sometimes relying too heavily on highly specialized jargon (Neimeyer, 1997). This has resulted in constructive therapies

https://doi.org/10.1037/0000468-005
Constructive Psychotherapies, by J. D. Raskin
Copyright © 2025 by the American Psychological Association. All rights reserved.

often seeming inaccessible to newcomers, which is unfortunate because—as previous chapters make clear—constructive therapies offer practical and concrete interventions despite the perception that they are obtuse, relativistic, and overly philosophical. This chapter addresses these two challenges by sharing the empirical evidence for constructive therapies as well as outlining and responding to common criticisms of constructive approaches.

EFFICACY

One way to evaluate constructive therapies is by examining research on their effectiveness. Although constructive therapists have done their fair share of randomized controlled experiments (Feixas et al., 2016; Feixas & Compañ, 2016; Karibwende et al., 2022; Paz et al., 2020; Pinheiro et al., 2014; Sun et al., 2022), they are hesitant about overemphasizing those experiments as well as the therapy manuals they often give rise to (Bohart et al., 1998; Botella, 2000; Marquis & Douthit, 2006; Procter & Winter, 2020). As part of ongoing efforts to sway "traditional" colleagues toward a more inclusive definition of evidence, constructive researchers stress methodological diversity, using both quantitative and qualitative methods to evaluate their interventions (Bridges & Raskin, in press). In this regard, constructive therapists align themselves with humanistic, feminist, and systemic colleagues who challenge the idea that experimental research is always preferable to other forms of inquiry.

For better or worse, constructive and other therapies that do not emphasize concrete techniques and medical model conceptualizations are more difficult to research via traditional experimental means (Bohart et al., 1998). These therapies are done a disservice when researchers dismiss alternative methods for studying them. This unfairly restricts what counts as evidence—and thereby disenfranchises these approaches (Bohart et al., 1998; Marquis & Douthit, 2006). In other words, "the therapies that are most likely to be 'empirically violated' or 'disenfranchised' in a naturalistic climate of empirical validation are constructivist, humanistic, and systemic approaches" (Procter & Winter, 2020, p. 279). Methodological pluralism militates against the marginalization of constructive therapies.

Another way to evaluate constructive therapies is by reviewing theoretical objections lodged against them. Constructive theories have been critiqued on a variety of grounds. The most prominent and well-known argument is that they espouse an antirealist relativism that inhibits therapeutic effectiveness by preventing constructive clinicians from making firm assertions or taking clear stands (Held, 1995, 1998; Mackay, 2011). This chapter evaluates research evidence for constructive therapies and responds to major critiques of constructive theory and practice.

Personal Construct Therapy

From its earliest days, personal construct therapy has been the subject of empirical research into its effectiveness (Markley et al., 1982; Procter & Winter, 2020). Experimental and case studies have been conducted on using personal construct therapy for a wide range of presenting complaints, including social anxiety and agoraphobia as well as other phobias and anxiety disorders (Beail & Parker, 1991; Lira et al., 1975; Paz et al., 2016; Winter et al., 2006). In addition, depression and related mood problems, such as fibromyalgia and postpartum depression (Domenici, 2007; Feixas et al., 2016; Paz et al., 2020; Pinheiro et al., 2014; Sheehan, 1985), eating disorders (Button, 1987), psychosis (Bannister et al., 1975), self-harm (Winter et al., 2007), sexual abuse (P. C. Alexander et al., 1989, 1991), stuttering (T. Stewart & Birdsall, 2001), and mental distress in breast cancer survivors (Lane & Viney, 2005, 2006), have all been investigated. Further, in an outcome study on diagnostically heterogeneous clients, personal construct therapy compared favorably with cognitive behavior therapy (CBT) and psychodynamic therapy (Watson & Winter, 2005). Although only a few of the studies cited here are randomized controlled experiments, they collectively suggest that personal construct therapy can be effective for a variety of therapeutic issues.

Fixed-role therapy, the one specific personal construct therapy technique that George Kelly (1955a, 1973) outlined, has been examined for use with forensic clients (Horley, 2006), people suffering from paraphilias (Horley, 2005), and individuals experiencing social anxiety (Iglesias &

Iglesias, 2014). Most of the investigations into fixed-role therapy have been case studies, including several conducted back in the 1940s while Kelly was developing his theory (Markley et al., 1982). The small body of existing evidence supports the continued use and development of fixed-role therapy.

In terms of general effectiveness, a 2006 meta-analysis suggested that personal construct therapy is more effective than no treatment, standard care, or being in a wait-list control group (Viney et al., 2006). This is consistent with the findings of systematic research reviews assessing personal construct therapy's overall effectiveness (Metcalfe et al., 2007; Winter, 1992, 2003)—although one more recent review found somewhat weaker efficacy for personal construct therapy than earlier reviews (J. M. Holland et al., 2007). Nonetheless, there appear to be modest but reliable effects for personal construct therapy across a variety of presenting problems (J. M. Holland & Neimeyer, 2009). Like many other approaches, personal construct therapy shows the largest effect sizes when used to treat fear and anxiety (J. M. Holland & Neimeyer, 2009). It has small to medium effects in treating stress and trauma, physical problems and aging, and problematic behavior (J. M. Holland & Neimeyer, 2009). Understandably, it is least effective for psychosis and delusional behavior (J. M. Holland & Neimeyer, 2009). See Figure 5.1 for a visual representation of these effects.

Narrative Therapy

The evidence base for narrative therapy is steadily growing but still in its early stages. There is an emerging body of evidence for the efficacy of narrative therapy with children. Narrative therapy has been found to be effective in improving social, emotional, and relationship skills among 8- to 10-year-old school children (Beaudoin et al., 2016, 2017). It also has shown promise in work with certain childhood populations. Evidence points to it reducing stress in 10- to 16-year-old children diagnosed with autism (Cashin et al., 2013), decreasing anxiety in children with imprisoned parents (Jalali et al., 2019), and increasing resilience in orphaned or abandoned children (Karibwende et al., 2022). Additional studies have found narrative therapy successfully reduced social phobia

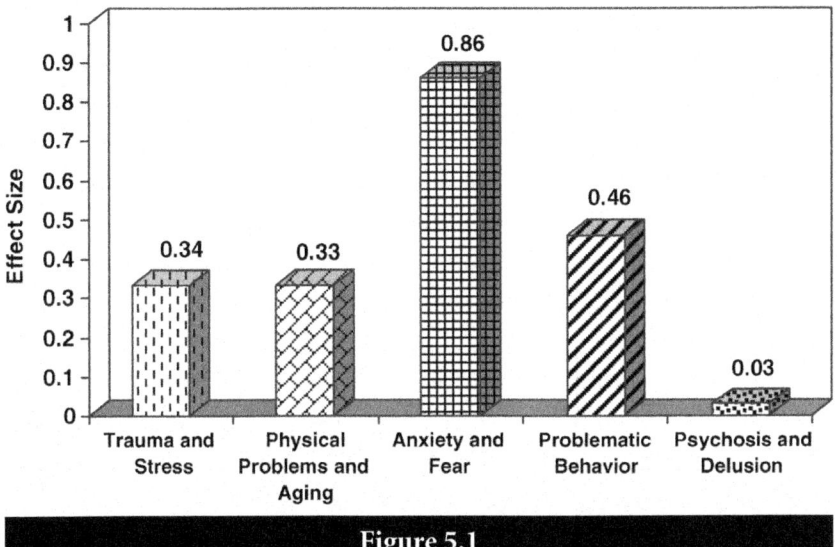

Figure 5.1

Note. Mean effect sizes for personal construct therapy (PCT) versus no active treatment comparisons across different types of presenting problems. From "The Efficacy of Personal Construct Therapy as a Function of the Type and Severity of the Presenting Problem," by J. M. Holland and R. A. Neimeyer, 2009, *Journal of Constructivist Psychology*, 22(2), p. 178 (https://doi.org/10.1080/10720530802675904). Copyright 2009 by Taylor and Francis. Reprinted with permission.

among boys (Looyeh et al., 2014), attention-deficit/hyperactivity disorder symptoms among girls (Looyeh et al., 2012), and mental health symptoms among adolescents in a juvenile boot camp (Ikonomopoulos et al., 2015). Although promising, many of these studies have small sample sizes, and most of them are not RCTs. Nonetheless, their results suggest that narrative therapy can benefit children facing a variety of challenging circumstances.

Beyond studies of children, research also supports the use of narrative therapy for specific presenting problems. Several studies have pointed to the efficacy of narrative therapy for mood disorders among both adults and children (Hawke et al., 2023; Jalali et al., 2019; Vromans & Schweitzer, 2011). Some of the research on mood disorders has suggested that narrative approaches are as effective as CBT (Lopes, Gonçalves, Fassnacht, et al.,

2014; Lopes, Gonçalves, Machado, et al., 2014). Narrative therapy has also been found efficacious in improving sexual functioning among women with skin cancer (Fallah & Ghodsi, 2022), in reducing stigma among patients with oral cancer (Sun et al., 2022), and in decreasing symptoms among women traumatized by sexual violence (Rani et al., 2024). It also has shown promise for treating those diagnosed with obsessive-compulsive disorder (Esfahani et al., 2015; Ghavibazou et al., 2022).

Despite these encouraging results, the evidence base for narrative therapy remains preliminary (Conti et al., 2022). Nonetheless, there are some presenting problems for which narrative therapy research is more voluminous. For example, studies have found narrative therapy to be a promising intervention for eating disorders and body dysmorphia (Heywood et al., 2022; Nagizadeh-Alamdari & Smkhani-Akbarinejhad, 2022).

Coherence Therapy and Narrative Solutions Therapy

There is very little published research on coherence therapy or narrative solutions therapy. This is not surprising because both are lesser known constructive approaches developed by practicing clinicians who were not working in research settings. Nevertheless, the model of change used in coherence therapy integrates findings from memory consolidation research (Ecker & Bridges, 2020). This body of research examines how new learning alters past learning.

The results of these investigations suggested that "new learning experiences directly revise existing contents of memory acquired in prior learning" (Ecker & Bridges, 2020, p. 287). Based on the findings of memory consolidation research, coherence therapists view their approach as incorporating the *empirically confirmed process of erasure*: Existing constructed memories are "erased" and replaced with new ones. Although memory consolidation research lends empirical support to the theory of coherence therapy, studies focused more directly on the effectiveness of coherence therapy and narrative solutions therapy would make important contributions to the therapy literature.

Context-Centered Therapy

Like coherence therapy and narrative solutions therapy, research on context-centered therapy remains scarce. However, one study did investigate a context-centered group treatment for social anxiety (Efran & Nath, 2004). The treatment entailed either two, 7-hour sessions held 1 week apart or four, 3½-hour sessions conducted over 2 weeks. The sessions incorporated context-centered therapy concepts such as "mind" and "self" and the notion that life is not personal. Results found that the treatment significantly decreased symptoms of social anxiety, including fear of negative evaluation, interpersonal sensitivity, and depression (Efran & Nath, 2004). These improvements were by and large sustained at a 6-month follow-up (Efran & Nath, 2004). Clearly, additional research on context-centered therapy is sorely needed.

Innovative Moments

One of the more groundbreaking and generative approaches to researching the effectiveness of constructive (and other) therapies is the innovative moments coding system (IMCS; Batista et al., 2020; Gonçalves et al., 2011). Unlike most therapy research, the *IMCS* approach is explicitly grounded in a constructive epistemology (Gonçalves et al., 2009, 2011). Its theoretical inspiration emerges from narrative therapy's previously discussed notion of unique outcomes—those commonly overlooked instances that contradict clients' dominant stories and meaning frameworks (Batista et al., 2020). In the narrowest sense, the term *innovative moments* (IMs) serves as a synonym for the narrative therapy notion of unique outcomes—this phrase having introduced two conceptual confusions because unique outcomes are neither unique (they happen all the time) nor what therapy researchers typically label outcomes (they reflect therapy process; Matos et al., 2009). More broadly, however, IMs occur whenever problem-causing patterns of functioning are disrupted and new patterns begin to emerge (Gonçalves et al., 2011). For example, a highly self-critical client encounters IMs any time they momentarily appreciate themselves or make sense of their experience in unfamiliar ways (Gonçalves et al., 2011).

IM research examines the relationship between IMs and therapeutic change. It explores links between IMs and the reconstruction of *problematic self-narratives*, defined as "implicit rules of meaning that constrain people's lives, strengths, or resources" (Montesano et al., 2017, p. 83). Because IMs are exceptions to problematic self-narratives, IMs researchers hypothesize that these moments are crucial to helping clients replace problematic narratives with more adaptive ones.

Research on IMs uses the IMCS to identify three different levels of IMs (Batista et al., 2020):

- *Level 1 IMs* are preliminary and "low-level" efforts at change that involve distancing or detaching from the problem (e.g., being aware of the effects of the problem, developing new strategies for overcoming the problem, reconsidering the causes of the problem).
- *Level 2 IMs* reflect "high-level" efforts at change that emphasize elaborating and expanding on Level 1 changes (e.g., investing in new relationships, developing new skills, making new meanings to explain what is changing).
- *Level 3 IMs* involve integrating and fully articulating new meanings (e.g., being able to explain what has changed, why it has changed, and how it has changed).

Research using the IMCS investigates connections between these three levels of IMs and psychotherapeutic change. This research involves training coders to identify different levels of IMs and then analyzing relationships between IMs and clinical outcomes. To date studies on IMs have consistently supported the hypothesis that IMs predict positive therapy outcomes and are fundamental to therapeutic change (Montesano et al., 2017). For instance, early research examining IMs in narrative therapy found that the occurrence of IMs predicts good outcomes, whereas their absence predicts poor outcomes (Cunha et al., 2012; Matos et al., 2009; Santos et al., 2011). More recent research on IMs has expanded its scope, finding that IMs predict better outcomes in a variety of therapeutic modalities, including psychodynamic, cognitive behavior, humanistic, brief-integrative, and transdiagnostic approaches (Drüge et al., 2023; Gonçalves et al., 2022; Nasim et al., 2019, 2021; Piazza-Bonin, Neimeyer, Alves, & Smigelsky, 2016; Piazza-Bonin, Neimeyer, Alves, Smigelsky, & Crunk, 2016; Sheena et al., 2024). Further, a growing collection of studies has linked IMs to the effectiveness of group therapy (Esposito et al., 2020, 2022, 2024; Garcia-Martínez et al., 2021; McGuinty et al., 2018). Across these different therapy modalities, the presence of IMs predicts clinical improvement for a variety of presenting complaints, including depression, anxiety, bereavement, grief, and bulimia (Alves et al., 2012; Batista et al., 2019; Cunha et al., 2012; Drüge et al., 2023; Fernández-Navarro et al., 2018, 2020; Gonçalves et al., 2016, 2022; Koutoufa et al., 2024; McGuinty et al., 2018; Mende et al., 2024; Piazza-Bonin, Neimeyer, Alves, & Smigelsky, 2016; Piazza-Bonin, Neimeyer, Alves, Smigelsky, & Crunk, 2016).

Taken as a whole, research on IMs suggests that the secret to effective therapy, regardless of theoretical orientation, is to provoke meaning reconstruction by upending status-quo narratives. Such research seamlessly integrates quantitative and qualitative methods without privileging RCTs over other approaches. In so doing, it offers an original and promising method to study therapeutic effectiveness—one that remains theoretically consistent with a constructive epistemology.

CRITICISMS

Constructive approaches have been criticized for denying reality and fostering an "anything goes" antirealism (Cobern & Loving, 2008; Held, 1995, 1998; Mackay, 2003, 2011; Martínez-Delgado, 2002). Further, they are often perceived as too theoretical and philosophical for everyday therapists to understand and appreciate (Neimeyer, 1997; Raskin, 2015). These two concerns about constructive therapies are examined and responded to next.

Undone by "Anything Goes" Antirealism

Anything Goes may be a lovely musical (Porter, 1934), but it is generally considered a terrible stance for those aspiring to scientific legitimacy. Unfortunately for constructive therapists, they have long been accused of espousing an "anything goes" antirealism that denies the existence of a stable external reality (Cobern & Loving, 2008; Held, 1995, 1998; Mackay, 2003, 2011; Martínez-Delgado, 2002). Critics have contended that constructive perspectives are dangerous because their antirealism "precludes any access—i.e., either a direct access (one not mediated by theory) or an indirect access (one mediated by theory)—to an independent reality" (Held, 1998, p. 199). This allegedly makes the constructive stance on therapeutic change untenable. Constructive therapy critics have argued that encouraging clients to change how they construe events is hazardous if it does not consider whether these revised constructions are true or not (Held, 1995, 1998). Changing one's constructions, these detractors warned, does not change reality. They further argued that the relativistic antirealism of constructive therapies produces theoretical incoherence: By adhering to the view that reality is constructed so that people are free to reconstrue it however they wish, constructive therapists presumably relinquish their ability to make truth claims—either about their clients' predicaments or their own theoretical perspective (Held, 1995, 1998).

Obviously, constructive therapists do not see themselves reflected in this caricature of their perspective. They challenge portrayals of them as "anything goes" relativists by rejecting the all-or-none notion of antirealism put forward by their critics (Efran & Heffner, 1998; Neimeyer, 1995; Raskin, 2001; Raskin & Debany, 2018). Asserting that people never know the world directly is not the same as saying there is no reality beyond our constructions of it. Recall from Chapter 3 the distinction between ontological and epistemological modes of construing. When construing ontologically, we accept the existence of a real world and assume that our constructions reflect our best efforts to map it. Even if these constructions are considered imperfect depictions of a world that can never be known directly or completely, this does not preclude believing in an external reality. From an integrative constructive stance, whenever one construes ontologically, it becomes perfectly reasonable to assume that our constructions reference an outside world (Raskin & Debany, 2018):

> Often it is necessary to preempt some constructions as true reflections of the real in order to get on with business. If a rock is hurtling

toward us, we will construe it ontologically as real, hard, and potentially dangerous. To do otherwise would be foolish. (Raskin & Debany, 2018, p. 348)

At the same time, constructive perspectives see no reason people must always construe ontologically. In some instances, shifting to an epistemological mode of construing in which we dismantle and challenge ideas about what we can and do know illuminates new and expansive possibilities: "Focusing on how and why people come to construe rocks—or, more interestingly for psychologists and counselors, human relationships—in particular ways profits from an epistemological mode of construing" (Raskin & Debany, 2018, p. 348). This recalls George Kelly's (1964/1969b) famous discussion about construing the floor as hard. When wishing to cross the room, construing the floor as hard and our construction of it as echoing reality works brilliantly. However, if one is a physicist studying the floor's particles microscopically, shifting to an epistemological mode of construing and questioning the ontological status of the floor as hard may be more fruitful (Raskin, 2011).

Constructive therapists maintain that too much reverence for the presumed correspondence between a real world and our meaning-making about it is not always in our best interest. Although fluctuating between the realism of ontological construing and the idealism of epistemological construing may run counter to traditional ideas about epistemology and psychotherapy, it is precisely what gives constructive therapies their unique "leverage." Encouraging clients to question their constructions of reality is the key ingredient of constructive therapies.

Mired in "Epistobabble"

As discussed throughout this volume, constructive therapy is a hands-on and an action-oriented approach in which clients examine their own constructed assumptions and then devise and test new ones. The goal is to foster new ways of client construing and behaving. Unfortunately, these pragmatic underpinnings of constructive therapy are often obscured by the abstractness of the corresponding literature. Constructive therapist

Robert Neimeyer (1997) lamented this, complaining that constructive therapies are too often mired in *epistobabble*—"terms, phrases and culture specific references to describe and create meaning within a social group with little attention to how others who may not have the requisite knowledge or background are affected" (Raskin et al., 2015, p. 302). Reflecting on constructive therapy, Neimeyer (1997) observed that "the abstract level at which constructivist discourse is typically pitched represents both boon and bane to this emerging tradition" (p. 53). Newcomers to constructive therapy encounter a daunting lexicon of befuddling terms, including "*constructive alternativism, second order cybernetics, autopoietic entities, narrative deconstruction, subjugated knowledges,* and *morphogenic nuclear structure*" (Neimeyer, 1997, p. 53). This dizzying array of strange terms

> can prove daunting to the psychotherapy practitioner, not to mention the beleaguered graduate student who trudges through courses in history and systems of psychology only to wade into still murkier waters upon embarking on coursework in the applied area of psychotherapy! (Neimeyer, 1997, p. 53)

It can be difficult to translate constructive therapy's alien and theoretically abstract terminology into clinical practice, and constructive therapists have not always done a good job explaining how to do so. This has created a significant obstacle to therapists interested in working constructively. Without clear illustrations of how to practice constructively, the utility of constructive therapies often goes unrecognized. It is hoped that this volume helps remedy this problem by providing a multitude of concrete examples while eschewing overreliance on opaque jargon.

6

Future Directions

In the world of unknowns, seek experience, and seek it full cycle.
—George A. Kelly (1977, p. 19)

Anticipation is a central idea in constructive therapies. People devise constructions to anticipate the future, then seek experience to test these constructions (Glasersfeld, 1984, 1995; Kelly, 1955a, 1969d, 1970). How can we anticipate what the future holds for constructive therapies? What predictions might we make? This chapter anticipates the future for constructive therapies by proposing several hypotheses. Time will tell whether these predictions come to pass.

https://doi.org/10.1037/0000468-006
Constructive Psychotherapies, by J. D. Raskin
Copyright © 2025 by the American Psychological Association. All rights reserved.

CONSTRUCTIVE PSYCHOTHERAPIES: HAMPERED BY SOME WORLD VIEWS, HELPED BY OTHERS

Pepper's (1942/1970) *root metaphor theory* holds that experiential reality is deeply influenced by the root metaphors we use to understand the world, and it proposes six metaphorical world views that shape human knowledge. Pepper (1942/1970) judged two of these world views (animism and mysticism) inadequate but held up the remaining four (formism, mechanism, contextualism, and organicism) as useful in understanding the world despite each yielding a different way to comprehend the nature of reality (Berry, 1984; Lyddon, 1989, 1995; Pepper, 1942/1970). All four of these world views have influenced psychotherapy generally and constructive therapies specifically—and I predict that they will continue to do so in the future. Let us briefly examine how.

Hampered by Formism and Mechanism

I predict that the commitment of many clinicians to two of Pepper's root metaphors, formism and mechanism, will continue to hamper constructive therapies. *Formism* relies on observed similarities in form, shape, or character to organize knowledge (Berry, 1984; Lyddon, 1989, 1995; Pepper, 1942/1970). For example, a square cardboard box and a Rubik's Cube share the same shape. Therefore, from a formistic perspective, they naturally go together. In a more psychological vein, formism groups people into "types" that share like characteristics. As an example, we might characterize two people—one fearful of heights and the other worried about social rejection—as both suffering from anxiety disorders.

Mechanism offers a different yet complementary metaphor. It assumes that the world can be understood by dividing it into components (Berry, 1984; Lyddon, 1989, 1995; Pepper, 1942/1970). For instance, taking apart a cuckoo clock can help us understand how it operates; the movement of its interlocking gears causes its hands to rotate and, when those hands strike 12, the cuckoo pops out, and chimes play. Shifting to a more psychological example, classic psychoanalytic theory (Freud, 1923/1960, 1933/1965) offers a mechanistic explanation of human behavior by contending that the distribution of psychic energy across the mental structures of id, ego, and superego determines personality (Lyddon, 1989). Analogously, cognitive therapies posit that irrational cognitions cause emotional upset: "The nature of an individual's beliefs about certain life events—namely, their degree of rationality, objectivity, or validity—are presumed to determine in a linear fashion his or her emotional adjustment" (Lyddon, 1989, p. 444).

Formism and mechanism dominate the psychological landscape yet are difficult to square with a constructive orientation. For instance, the explanatory power of trait-based taxonomies, such as the Big Five personality model (McCrae, 2017; McCrae & Costa, 1997; McCrae & John, 1992), and psychiatric nosologies, such as the American Psychiatric Association's (2022) *Diagnostic and Statistical Manual of Mental Disorders* (5th ed., text rev.; *DSM-5-TR*) and the World Health Organization's (2019) *International Classification of Diseases and Related Health Problems* (11th ed.; *ICD-11*), rest on formistic and mechanistic foundations. The Big Five model assumes that "personal characteristics are primary determinants of psychological functioning" (Lyddon, 1989, p. 443). As such, it implicitly embraces both formism (people have measurable and distinct "traits" that we can recognize based on their similarities) and mechanism (these traits cause people's thoughts, feelings, and actions). Similarly, the *DSM-5-TR* and *ICD-11* assume "that certain classes of relatively stable psychological disorders exist and that these disorders may be differentiated from one another on the basis of like and unlike features (symptoms)" (Lyddon, 1989, pp. 443–444). Here again, we see the influence of formism (similar constellations of behavior represent similar forms of psychological disorder) and mechanism (these disorders cause people's symptoms). Thus, we can construe the Big Five, *DSM-5-TR*, and *ICD-11* as exemplars of formism and mechanism.

Formistic and mechanistic perspectives will remain influential in the field of psychotherapy for the near future; the Big Five, *DSM-5-TR*, and *ICD-11* are not going anywhere anytime soon because they fit too well with unquestioned assumptions about people having "essential personalities" that can be parsed into diagnostic "types." This situation poses challenges for constructive therapists, who often regard formism and mechanism with suspicion. They are skeptical of formism because they see it as reflecting therapist, not client, meaning-making. The Big Five, *DSM-5-TR*, and *ICD-11* tell us about how therapists construe clients, not how clients construe themselves and the world. Constructive therapists are interested in understanding their clients' unique and individualized personal meanings, not in categorizing their clients using therapist-derived trait or symptom groupings. This is their rationale for using idiographic assessments, such as the rep grid (Fromm, 2004; Jankowicz, 2003; Procter & Winter, 2020). Further, constructive therapists tend to see people as active and agentic meaning-makers (Kelly, 1955a, 1955b). Consequently, they question mechanistic models that reduce human psychology to a set of presumed causal components (Leitner & Faidley, 2002; Raskin & Epting, 1993).

Suspicion of formistic and mechanistic models in psychotherapy has implications for the future of constructive therapies. It places constructive therapists at odds with dominant views in the field. Thus, constructive therapists may continue to find themselves outside the mainstream, along with like-minded humanistic and feminist colleagues who also question the dominance of formist and mechanist world views (Bohart et al., 1998; L. S. Brown, 2000, 2018; Kamens et al., 2017). To avoid marginalization, constructive clinicians must continue pointing out that their approach to assessment and diagnosis—with its emphasis on individual meanings rather than diagnostic and trait pigeonholes—only seems out of step if one remains committed to formistic and mechanistic perspectives. This is an uphill battle, and one likely to continue in the years ahead. It involves pushing back against the dominant medical model that attributes mental distress to "disorders" people "have" while highlighting how individual and collaborative meaning-making can focus on taken-for-granted beliefs and practices (both individual and social) that perpetuate human suffering.

Helped by the Rise of Contextualism and Organicism

Although constructive therapies will be hampered by the continued influence of formism and mechanism, I also predict that they will be helped by the mental health professions' increasing reliance on Pepper's (1942/1970) contextualist and organicist metaphors. *Contextualism* presumes that events and their surroundings are inextricably intertwined historical events that mutually influence one another (Berry, 1984; Lyddon, 1989, 1995; Pepper, 1942/1970). From a contextualist perspective, everything that occurs does so within a context. For example, a ball can only be "fair" or "foul" within the context of baseball. Similarly, one can only be a "patron" or "server" within the context of "restaurants" or a "therapist" or "patient" within the context of "psychotherapy." In other words, human experience must be understood in context. The *reciprocal determinism* of contextualist approaches requires moving beyond unidirectional causal connections (Lyddon, 1989, 1995). No one factor singularly determines all others. Instead, multiple factors (e.g., genes, environment, cognitions, behaviors) mutually influence one another in an ongoing, process-oriented manner (Lyddon, 1989, 1995).

Organicism holds that an organized set of dynamic processes underlie the development of all phenomena (Berry, 1984; Lyddon, 1989, 1995; Pepper, 1942/1970). In biology, an organicist metaphor helps us understand the metamorphosis of a mealworm from larva to pupa to adult beetle. In psychology, the notion of people as dynamic and ever-changing systems forever "in process" also reflects the organicist perspective (Maturana & Varela, 1992); "personal growth" is an ongoing process that continuously unfolds throughout life. Correspondingly, the shift in emphasis among psychotherapy researchers from outcomes to process similarly reflects an organicist world view (Lyddon, 1989; Wampold & Imel, 2015). From the perspective of organicism, only by understanding moment-to-moment occurrences in the consulting room can we comprehend the ongoing evolution of human change processes (Mahoney, 1991).

Constructive therapies lean heavily on contextualist and organicist metaphors. Although context-centered therapy is most explicitly contextualist (the word "context" is in its name!), all constructive therapies emphasize context in understanding client dilemmas. The meanings people devise always occur at specific times and places. They are simultaneously products of personal and social processes and pressures that can never be completely disentangled. As such, they forever influence and determine one another.

There seems to be an increasing emphasis on contextualism and organicism in psychotherapy circles. The rise of multicultural perspectives in counseling and psychotherapy exemplifies and fosters this shift (American Psychological Association, 2017; Vasquez & Johnson, 2022). Cultural context matters. This seems obvious to therapists today, but it is only over the past 3 decades or so that multicultural counseling has come into its own. Although no longer as popular as it was in the 1970s and 1980s, systems theory (Bertalanffy, 1972/1972; Bowen, 1978; Doherty & McDaniel, 2009; Minuchin, 1974; Mitchell, n.d.; Steinglass, 1984) offers another organicist approach with connections to constructive therapies. In the years ahead, constructive therapies will benefit from there being a large cohort of therapists—multicultural, systems, and beyond—who are grounded in and committed to contextual and organicist world views.

WHAT ABOUT TRAINING OPPORTUNITIES?

On a very practical level, one of the challenges facing constructive therapies is whether adequate training opportunities will be available to practitioners interested in them. Many graduate training programs provide a cursory introduction to constructive therapies, but in-depth training opportunities are more difficult to find. An exception is the University of Padua in Italy, which provides extensive training in personal construct therapy. Its first-level university master's program, offered in conjunction with the University of Hertfordshire in the United Kingdom, is a 2-year online program that trains students in the theory and practice of personal construct psychology and counseling. Alternatively, the School of Constructivist Psychotherapy at the Institute of Constructivist Psychotherapy—also in Padua—offers a 4-year course of study in constructivist therapies; its curriculum includes training in individual, couples, family, and group modalities along with training in organizational counseling and consultation. The *Centro Studi in Psicoterapia Cognitiva Costruttivista* [Center for Studies in Cognitive Constructivist Psychotherapy] in Florence, Italy, houses a specialization in constructivist psychotherapy. Outside of Italy, the University of Barcelona in Spain administers a master's degree certificate in cognitive and social therapy with a focus on constructivist and systems perspectives, whereas the United Kingdom is home to the Coventry Constructivist Centre, which offers a diploma course and related training opportunities. If one is looking for training in narrative therapy, in Australia, the Dulwich Center in Adelaide delivers online courses, 1-week intensives, a 1-year training program, and a master in narrative therapy in conjunction with the University of Melbourne.

Although fewer constructive therapy training programs are available in the United States, motivated clinicians still have several options. Those interested in constructive therapy approaches to grief and loss can earn training certificates at the Portland Institute for Loss and Transition. Further, the Coherence Psychology Institute in New York City provides short online courses, certificate programs, and case consultation services in coherence therapy. For those interested in narrative therapy, the Vancouver School for Narrative Therapy offers both certificate and continuing education programs, whereas the Narrative Therapy Initiative offers a variety of online trainings and case consultations. In a similar vein, the Taos Institute runs a diploma program in social construction and professional practice along with related workshops, online courses, and certificate programs.

Those seeking something a bit less intensive can find various continuing education classes and training videos on constructive psychotherapies online (see https://alexanderstreet.com). The future of constructive therapies will hinge on the continued availability of these training opportunities and the establishment of others. See the Suggested Readings and Resources section at the end of this volume for further details on training in constructive therapies.

7

Summary

It's in the way that you use it.
—Eric Clapton (1986, Line 1)

In keeping with their philosophical pragmatism, constructive therapists view theories of psychotherapy as useful tools, not ultimate truths. Constructive clinicians select the therapeutic theories and techniques that they predict will allow them to best conceptualize and assist the client at hand. When they find a theoretical approach and its implications beneficial, they use it. However, when a conceptualization falls flat, constructive therapists feel no compunction about trading it for a better alternative. In this respect, constructive clinicians do not treat theories of therapy (even their own) with too much reverence. They treat them as conjectures to be used when they work and discarded when they do not. This permits a refreshing degree of clinical openness and flexibility.

The pragmatic spirit of constructive theories has informed the development of this volume. As noted in Chapter 5, previous overviews of constructive therapies were often long on theory but light on practice. This has hindered appreciation of the highly practical and hands-on nature of constructive interventions. The goal of this book has been to illustrate that constructive therapies do indeed offer concrete and easy-to-use clinical strategies, such as those outlined in Chapter 4. Moreover, contrary to common belief, implementing these strategies does not require a background in philosophy or epistemology. All the abstract theorizing that surrounds (and often confounds comprehension of) constructive therapies revolves around one simple yet revolutionary idea: that people experience life through frameworks of meaning that they create for themselves—both singly and collectively. In other words, constructive clinicians maintain that people never know the world in its totality or in a manner that perfectly reflects reality. This simple assertion has profound implications in many areas of inquiry, but herein, we have mainly concerned ourselves with its effect on the conduct of psychotherapy. Changing clients' lives requires transforming their meaning-making because, from a constructive perspective, how people construe brings experiential realities into being; it informs what people take for granted as true.

This means that there is always diversity in how people construe events. However, for constructive therapists, diversity goes beyond a mere embrace of multiculturalism. Diversity means attending to how construing is informed not only by therapy clients' religious, ethnic, racial, socioeconomic, and cultural statuses but also by the uniqueness of their specific relationships and life histories. All these things combine to yield *each distinct client's individualized meaning-making.* Equally important, constructive therapies see the concepts that people use to organize their understanding of diversity (e.g., ethnicity, race, gender) as constructions that people have invented. Like all constructions conveyed via language, they have advantages and disadvantages. Just as with psychotherapy theories, therapists and clients are always at liberty to use, revise, or discard these constructions as they see fit. Reifying them is never required.

SUMMARY

Of course, avoiding reification can be difficult. Twentieth century American psychologist George Kelly, founder of personal construct psychology (and arguably the first modern constructive theorist and therapist), was painfully aware of how language reifies ideas:

> The subject-predicate form of our Indo-European languages has led us to confound objects with what is said about them. Thus every time we open our mouths to say something, we break forth with a dogmatism. Each sentence, instead of sounding like a proposal of an idea to be examined in the light of personal experience, echoes through the room like the disembodied rumblings of an oracle. (Kelly, 1958/1969c, p. 68)

Psychotherapy has been especially vulnerable to oraclelike rumblings. Those entering the field encounter a mind-numbing array of competing theories, each sporting a cadre of enthusiastic and vociferous proponents—true believers. Constructive therapies embrace Kelly's belief that all theories (including constructive ones) are humanly invented tools for understanding, rather than God's-eye reflections of truth itself. Theoretical assertions are "no more than partially accurate constructions of events" to "eventually be overthrown and displaced" (Kelly, 1958/1969c, p. 66). Thus, the goal of this book has not been to suggest that constructive approaches to therapy are correct in some sort of universal and eternal way. Rather, in keeping with the thoroughgoing pragmatism of constructive theories (Butt, 2000; McWilliams, 2016a), this book's ambitions have been more modest. Readers have been invited to consider the utility of constructive approaches—how they offer viable and well-supported frameworks for psychotherapy.

Frameworks are built by people. Therefore, constructive theories view all frameworks (again, even their own) as humanly invented templates devised to enhance understanding and guide action. With that key point in mind, the aim of this volume has been to provide a basic overview of constructive therapies. In Chapter 2, I outlined historical antecedents of modern constructive approaches, showing how constructive thought has long been embedded in the history of ideas, including (of course) psychology and psychotherapy. Chapter 3 fleshed out in greater detail the three main theories that inform constructive therapies: (a) personal constructivism, (b) radical constructivism, and (c) social constructionism. Therapeutic strategies that spring from these theories were presented in Chapter 4 along with case examples to illustrate these approaches. Chapter 5 summarized research support for constructive therapies. It also outlined common critiques of constructive perspectives and presented rejoinders to these criticisms. Chapter 6 discussed future directions for constructive therapies.

This chapter brings things to a close by reminding readers that constructive therapies—like all therapies, and all stories that clients share—are human inventions that provide tools for living life. Constructive therapists use these tools to help clients revise their constructions, thereby alleviating mental distress.

Constructive therapies have a great deal to offer both experienced and budding clinicians. These therapies provide a way to make sense of client problems that uniquely balances insight and action. Clients gain insight when they become aware of the taken-for-granted ways that they construe their lives. Yet, constructive therapies move beyond merely talk; they also stress and encourage action. Viewing behavior as an experiment, constructive therapists invite clients to do something differently to explore novel possibilities. The results can prove transformative, opening new and unanticipated ways to meaningfully experience self, others, and world. Insight and action together constitute the fundamentals of change.

Constructive therapies are ideal for therapists who like to innovate. Therapists who prefer creative to doctrinaire or scripted interventions are most likely to find themselves drawn to constructive perspectives. Although certain clinical strategies work with many clients, therapy must always be tailored and adapted to the client at hand. In this regard, constructive therapists view therapy similarly to how Heraclitus, the ancient Greek philosopher discussed in Chapter 2, viewed rivers: A person never steps into the same river twice. Likewise, a therapist never conducts the same therapy (or even the same session) twice. Every client is different and requires an original approach. No matter how many one-size-fits-all therapy manuals are devised, every therapy experience is unique. The constructive principle of orthogonal interaction holds that the key to therapeutic effectiveness is not doing the same thing repeatedly across clients. Rather, the linchpin of consistent clinical success is to idiosyncratically engage each client in a distinct manner that surprises and disrupts that specific client's individualized presuppositions about and orientation toward the world. This gives therapists a wide berth to think innovatively about their work. To reiterate, one never does therapy the same way twice.

Throughout the book, I have tried to present constructive therapies in a manner consistent with what George Kelly (1964/1969b) called the *invitational mood*, which invites clients to entertain alternative constructions without insisting that these constructions be viewed as once-and-for-all interpretations. This contrasts with the *indicative mood*, in which language is treated as indicating, in a final and inarguable way, how things are (Kelly, 1964/1969b). Like ontological mode construing (discussed in Chapters 2 and 5), the indicative mood has its place. However, it can limit imagination. Returning to the centrality of language in constituting experiential reality, constructive therapies suggest that changing how we construe and talk about events opens new possibilities. It lets us, as Kelly put it, "extricate ourselves from the kind of realism to which our so-called objective language system has bound us" (Kelly, 1964/1969b, p. 162). "Nowhere is this semantic enslavement clearer," Kelly (1964/1969b) concluded, "than in the psychotherapy room" (p. 162).

Glossary of Key Terms

ABC MODEL   Personal construct assessment technique that identifies how positive pole shifts on one construct have negative implications for pole shifts on other constructs.

COHERENCE THERAPY   A constructive therapy that combines the meaning-focus of personal construct therapy with neuroscience research on memory reconsolidation; focuses on implicit meanings that clients are not aware of but that provide compelling ways of understanding the world that necessitate presenting symptoms or problems.

CONSTRUCTIVE ALTERNATIVISM   Underlying premise of personal constructivism; holds that there are always alternative ways to understand the world and that all our interpretations of it are subject to revision or replacement.

CONSTRUCTIVE THEORIES   Theories contending that people and the social groups they form know the world indirectly through mental templates of their own creation.

CONSTRUCTIVE THERAPIES   Therapies that disrupt and reinterpret clients' reified meanings and thereby initiate reconstruction processes that open new possibilities.

CONTEXT-CENTERED THERAPY   Therapy that provokes client change through the identification and shifting of the humanly constructed contexts that shape experience.

CONTEXTS   Sets of humanly devised assumptions that frame and organize experience.

CONTEXTUALISM   One of Stephen C. Pepper's root metaphors for knowledge; presumes that events and their surroundings are inextricably intertwined historical events that mutually influence one another.

CORE CONSTRUCTS   In personal construct psychology, the constructs most important to a person and central to their sense of identity.

CREDULOUS APPROACH   In personal construct psychotherapy, a stance of openness and acceptance adopted by a clinician to understand how the client is presently experiencing the world.

DISCOURSES   Social constructionist term for the joint ways of talking and living that people use to collectively bring into being shared experiential realities.

EMPIRICALLY CONFIRMED PROCESS OF ERASURE (ECPE)   Relying on neuroscience research on memory; the assumption in coherence therapy that existing constructed memories are "erased" and replaced with new ones.

EPISTEMOLOGICAL CONSTRUING   Mode of construing that occurs whenever we shift from treating our constructions as ontological reflections of a presumed external world to viewing them as useful creations of our own making.

EPISTOBABBLE   Use of confusing and unclear theoretical and philosophical jargon related to epistemology; constructive theories are sometimes accused of overreliance on it.

EXCEPTIONS   In narrative therapy, instances when the problem had less of an influence over the client.

EXPERIENTIAL PERSONAL CONSTRUCT THERAPY   A variant of personal construct therapy that places the interpersonal aspects of construing—especially role relationships—front and center.

EXTERNALIZING THE PROBLEM   Narrative therapy technique in which clients are invited to view and talk about their problems as separate and distinct from (i.e., "external to") themselves.

FIXED-ROLE SKETCH   In fixed-role therapy, the sketch written in the third person of someone different from the client in important ways;

the client enacts the sketch, usually for 2 weeks, to experiment with new ways of behaving and construing.

FIXED-ROLE THERAPY   Personal construct therapy technique that has clients play roles that diverge in important ways from how they presently construe themselves; allows them to test new constructs in a nonthreatening way.

FORMISM   One of Stephen C. Pepper's root metaphors for knowledge; relies on observed similarities in form, shape, or character as a way to organize knowledge.

FOUR PREMISES OF AN INTEGRATED CONSTRUCTIVE PSYCHOLOGY   (a) people are informationally closed systems, only in direct contact with their own processes; (b) people are active meaning-makers, drawing distinctions as they construct ways of understanding; (c) people are social beings, using their intersubjective experiences to confirm the utility of their constructions; and (d) people engage in both ontological and epistemological modes of construing, alternating between them as necessary.

GAP   In narrative solutions therapy, the discrepancy between a person's preferred view and how others view that person or between a person's preferred view and behavior.

IMPLICATIONS GRID   Repertory grid technique that asks clients to rate the implications of changing poles on one of their constructs by checking off which of their other constructs they would also change poles on as a result.

INDICATIVE MOOD   Personal construct psychology term for describing when language is treated as indicating in a final and inarguable way how things are.

INFORMATIONALLY CLOSED SYSTEMS   Radical constructivist term describing how organisms are never directly in touch with the world itself and, instead, are only in touch with their own internal processes; information never gets in or out—rather, the world triggers internal meaning-making processes in the person, the results of which constitute knowledge.

INNOVATIVE MOMENTS (IM)   Preferred term used by innovative moment therapy researchers instead of the narrative therapy term *unique outcomes* (or *sparkling moments*); refers to times when the client has effectively avoided falling prey to the problem.

INNOVATIVE MOMENTS CODING SYSTEM (IMCS)   Coding system used in innovative moments research; uses various levels to classify moments of change in psychotherapy.

INTERSUBJECTIVE REALITY   Radical constructivist term for the experience of shared reality that results when others respond to us in a manner that confirms our sense that they understand things as we do—even though, according to radical constructivism, we are informationally closed systems never directly in touch with one another's personal and private meanings.

INVITATIONAL MOOD   Personal construct psychology term for inviting others to entertain alternative constructions without insisting that these constructions be viewed as once-and-for-all interpretations.

LADDERING   Personal construct assessment technique to elicit and explore the implications of client constructs, metaphorically climbing from lower level (*subordinate*) constructs to higher level (*superordinate*) ones that are more central and important to the client's world view.

MACROSOCIAL PROCESSES   Broad social discourses (e.g., "marriage," "fame," "romantic love") that frame and contextualize people's experiences—including their microsocial interactions.

MAPPING THE INFLUENCE OF THE PROBLEM   Narrative therapy technique in which clients are asked "mapping" questions about the externalized problem, such as: "What role does the problem have on your life?" "In what ways does the problem act like it's your friend when it's not?" "When are you most vulnerable to the influence of the problem?" and "Who in your life would be least surprised at your ability to stand up to the problem?"

MECHANISM   One of Stephen C. Pepper's root metaphors for knowledge; assumes that the world can be understood by dividing it into components.

MICROSOCIAL PROCESSES   In social constructionism, specific interactions among specific groups of two or more people.

MIND   In context-centered therapy, a context that narrowly frames the world in strictly defensive and self-protective terms; when operating from mind, people focus exclusively on winning, being right, and staying safe.

NARRATIVE SOLUTIONS THERAPY   Constructive therapy that integrates elements of personal construct therapy, solution-focused therapy, strategic therapy, and person-centered therapy; focuses on the link between mental distress and preferred view.

NARRATIVE THERAPY   Constructive therapy that contends that the stories people construct—alone and in concert with one another—are responsible for the psychological quagmires in which they find themselves.

NOMINAL FALLACIES   Occur when people mistake the names that they use to describe themselves for explanations of their behavior.

ONTOLOGICAL CONSTRUING   Mode of construing that presumes the existence of a world separate from one's understanding of it.

OPTIMAL THERAPEUTIC DISTANCE   Term in experiential personal construct therapy that indicates being close enough to clients to intimately experience their feelings but distant enough to recognize their feelings as distinct and separate from one's own.

ORGANICISM   One of Stephen C. Pepper's root metaphors for knowledge; holds that an organized set of dynamic processes underlie the development of all phenomena.

ORTHOGONAL INTERACTION   Occurs when someone responds to us differently than we are used to, eliciting novel reactions; important term in context-centered therapy.

PERSON AS DISCOURSE USER   Metaphor in social constructionism that sees people as actively internalizing and using socially constructed discourses to understand themselves and the world.

PERSON AS SCIENTIST   Metaphor in personal constrictivism that views people as personal scientists who actively form hypotheses and predict events.

PERSONAL CONSTRUCT   A dimension of psychological meaning consisting of something and its perceived opposite; each individual creates their own personal constructs.

PERSONAL CONSTRUCT THERAPY   Therapy that springs from 20th century psychologist George Kelly's personal construct theory.

PERSONAL CONSTRUCTIVISM   Constructive theory devised by 20th century psychologist George Kelly that holds that people devise private systems of psychological meanings made up of "personal constructs," each consisting of two "poles": the first being an idea and the second being its perceived opposite (also called *personal construct psychology* or *personal construct theory*).

PHILOLOGICAL CONSULTANT   Constructive term that describes what therapists do; the term implies that the therapist's role is as language expert who decodes and clarifies the meaning of client utterances.

PREFERRED VIEW   Narrative solutions therapy term for the way each of us prefers to see ourselves and prefers to be seen by others.

PREVERBAL CONSTRUING   In personal construct psychology, construing for which there are no words; underdeveloped, unspoken, and tacit meanings.

PROBLEM-SATURATED STORIES   Narrative therapy term for client narratives in which clients and their problems are fused, thereby pathologizing clients; problems are viewed as emanating from within people.

PYRAMIDING   Personal construct elicitation technique that, in contrast to laddering, "climbs down" the construct system from more central to less central constructs.

RADICAL CONSTRUCTIVISM   Term for the related but distinct constructive theories of Ernst von Glasersfeld and Humberto Maturana; these theories view people's experiential realities as stemming from a "structure determined" combination of biological and psychological processes.

RECIPROCAL DETERMINISM   No one factor singularly determines all others; instead, multiple factors (e.g., genes, environment, cognitions, behaviors) mutually influence one another in an ongoing, process-oriented manner.

REPERTORY GRID (REP GRID)   Assessment technique in personal constructivism used to elicit and measure people's unique personal constructs.

RESISTANCE TO CHANGE GRID   Repertory grid technique that explores client preferences for maintaining rather than shifting from preferred construct poles.

ROLE RELATIONSHIP   Term in personal constructivism for when two people construe each other's construction processes well enough to play roles in a social relationship together; role relationships are central to experiential personal construct therapy, whose adherents capitalize the word "role" ("ROLE relationships") to capture the deep and intimate way in which experiential personal construct psychotherapy conceptualizes roles.

ROOT METAPHOR THEORY   Stephen C. Pepper's theory that holds that experiential reality is deeply influenced by six root metaphors people use to understand the world; Pepper judged two of the worldviews that emerge from these metaphors (animism and mysticism) inadequate but held up the remaining four (formism, mechanism, contextualism, and organicism) as useful in understanding the world despite each yielding a different way to comprehend the nature of reality.

SELF   In context-centered therapy, a context that is broader than the context of mind because, instead of dwelling on safety and self-protection, its focus is on empathy, connection, and affinity with others.

SOCIAL CONSTRUCTIONISM   Constructive theory that says meaning is something people create together through their ongoing relationships; how people talk, interact, and communally coordinate with one another shapes shared social understanding.

SPARKLING MOMENTS   In narrative therapy, times when the client has effectively avoided falling prey to the externalized problem; sometimes called *unique outcomes*.

STRUCTURE DETERMINISM   Radical constructivist idea that the way an organism is built—its psychological and biological structures—constrains and shapes how it can perceive, respond, and know.

UNIQUE OUTCOMES   In narrative therapy, times when the client has effectively avoided falling prey to the externalized problem; sometimes called *sparkling moments*.

Suggested Readings and Resources

READINGS

Bannister, D., & Fransella, F. (2019). *Inquiring man: The psychology of personal constructs* (3rd ed.). Routledge. (Original work published 1986)

Chiari, G., & Nuzzo, M. L. (2010). *Constructivist psychotherapy: A narrative hermeneutic approach.* Routledge.

Ecker, B., & Hulley, L. (1996). *Depth-oriented brief therapy.* Jossey-Bass Publishers.

Ecker, B., & Hulley, L. (2008). Coherence therapy: Swift change at the core of emotional truth. In J. D. Raskin & S. K. Bridges (Eds.), *Studies in meaning 3: Constructivist psychotherapy in the real world* (pp. 57–84). Pace University Press.

Efran, J. S., Lukens, M. D., & Lukens, R. J. (1990). *Language, structure, and change: Frameworks of meaning in psychotherapy.* W. W. Norton & Co.

Epting, F. R. (1984). *Personal construct counseling and psychotherapy.* John Wiley & Sons.

Fromm, M. (2004). *Introduction to the repertory grid interview.* Waxmann Münster.

Glasersfeld, E. von. (1984). An introduction to radical constructivism. In P. Watzlawick (Ed.), *The invented reality: How do we know what we believe we know? Contributions to constructivism* (pp. 17–40). W. W. Norton & Company.

Glasersfeld, E. von. (1995). *Radical constructivism: A way of knowing and learning.* The Falmer Press.

Glasersfeld, E. von (2007). Aspects of constructivism: Vico, Berkeley, Piaget. In M. Larochelle (Ed.), *Key works in radical constructivism* (pp. 91–99). Sense Publishers. (Original work published 1992)

Jankowicz, D. (2003). *The easy guide to repertory grids.* Wiley.

SUGGESTED READINGS AND RESOURCES

Kelly, G. A. (1955a). *The psychology of personal constructs: Vol. 1. A theory of personality.* W. W. Norton.

Kelly, G. A. (1955b). *The psychology of personal constructs: Vol. 2. Clinical diagnosis and psychotherapy.* W. W. Norton.

Kelly, G. A. (1963). *A theory of personality: The psychology of personal constructs.* W. W. Norton.

Mahoney, M. J. (2003). *Constructive psychotherapy: A practical guide.* The Guilford Press.

Maturana, H. R., & Varela, F. J. (1992). *The tree of knowledge: The biological roots of human understanding* (Rev ed.; R. Paolucci, Trans.). Shambhala.

McNamee, S., Rasera, E. F., & Martins, P. (2023). *Practicing therapy as social construction.* SAGE Publishing.

Neimeyer, R. A. (2009). *Constructivist psychotherapy: Distinctive features.* Routledge.

Neimeyer, R. A., & Mahoney, M. J. (Eds.). (1995). *Constructivism in psychotherapy.* American Psychological Association. https://doi.org/10.1037/10170-000

Procter, H., & Winter, D. A. (2020). *Personal and relational construct psychotherapy.* Palgrave Macmillan. https://doi.org/10.1007/978-3-030-52177-6

Raskin, J. D., & Bridges, S. K. (2024). Constructivist theories in psychotherapy. In F. T. L. Leong, J. L. Callahan, J. Zimmerman, M. J. Constantino, & C. F. Eubanks (Eds.), *APA handbook of psychotherapy: Vol. 1. Theory-driven practice and disorder-driven practice* (pp. 257–272). American Psychological Association. https://doi.org/10.1037/0000353-015

Raskin, J. D., & Efran, J. S. (2020). The practice of context-centered therapy: A conversation with Jay S. Efran. *The Humanistic Psychologist, 48*(2), 202–219. https://doi.org/10.1037/hum0000143

VIDEOS

American Psychological Association. (2004, June). *Constructivist therapy: Robert A. Neimeyer, PhD* [Video]. https://www.apa.org/pubs/videos/4310704

American Psychological Association. (2008, May). *Constructivist therapy over time: Robert A. Neimeyer, PhD* [DVD]. https://www.apa.org/pubs/videos/4310849

American Psychological Association. (2022, January). *Engaging and connecting with clients online: Robert A. Neimeyer, PhD* [DVD]. https://www.apa.org/pubs/videos/engaging-connecting-clients-online

American Psychological Association. (2024, May). *Constructive therapy in practice: Jonathan D. Raskin, PhD* [DVD]. https://www.apa.org/pubs/videos/constructive-therapy-practice

Animas Centre for Coaching. (2023, December 12). *Constructivist foundations of coaching: A conversation with Dr. Jelena Pavlović* [Video]. YouTube. https://www.youtube.com/watch?v=T__hSNdlU6E

Bacon, S. (2021, August 8). *Social constructionism explains how therapy actually works* [Video]. YouTube. https://www.youtube.com/watch?v=nAyL_IKpMSQ

Gibbs, G. R. (2012a, October 30). *Personal constructs. Part 1 of 2 on personal construct psychology* [Video]. YouTube. https://www.youtube.com/watch?v=SeRv62ugJFc

Gibbs, G. R. (2012b, October 30). *The repertory grid. Part 2 of 2 on personal construct psychology* [Video]. YouTube. https://www.youtube.com/watch?v=YFlwtIaSxjo

Psychotherapy Expert Talks. (2016, July 24). *Robert A. Neimeyer on constructivist therapy and grief therapy* [Video]. YouTube. https://www.youtube.com/watch?v=tMX_1yeKNoI

Psychotherapy Networker. (2012, July 16). *Jay Efran: The emotion revolution excerpt* [Video]. YouTube. https://www.youtube.com/watch?v=pxPmvD_DwXE

Psychotherapy Networker. (2016, October 19). *VIDEO: Jay Efran on what to do when clients cry* [Video]. YouTube. https://www.youtube.com/watch?v=ErSPVL4N8yc

SHP-TV by The Society for Humanistic Psychology—APA Division 32. (2022, December 14). *Constructivist therapies: A brief introduction* [Video]. YouTube. https://www.youtube.com/watch?v=bclobG1oVcM

Sposini, F. M. (2014, April 17). *Ken Gergen talks about social constructionist ideas, theory and practice* [Video]. YouTube. https://www.youtube.com/watch?v=-AsKFFX9Ib0

ThinkPlay Partners. (2019, April 15). *Sheila McNamee—Relational engagement* [Video]. YouTube. https://www.youtube.com/watch?v=k0tAbIlgGAQ

TRAINING

- Coherence Psychology Institute: https://www.coherencetherapy.org/training/courses.htm
- Coventry Constructivist Centre: https://covpcp.com
- Dulwich Centre: https://dulwichcentre.com.au/
- Institute of Constructivist Psychology: https://www.icp-italia.it/it
- Lifelong Learning Master's Degree Certificate in Cognitive and Social Therapy: Constructivist and systemic training (University of Barcelona): https://web.ub.edu/en/web/estudis/w/specificmasterdegree-202311611?presentation

SUGGESTED READINGS AND RESOURCES

- Narrative Therapy Initiative: https://www.narrativetherapyinitiative.org/training-program
- Personal Construct Psychology Association: https://personalconstructuk.org
- Portland Institute for Loss and Transition: https://www.portlandinstitute.org
- School of Constructivist Psychotherapy at the Institute of Constructivist Psychology: https://www.icp-italia.it/en/the-school/the-school-of-constructivist-psychotherapy
- *Scuola di Specializzazione in Psicoterapia Costruttivista Intersoggettiva* [School of Specialization in Intersubjective Constructivist Psychotherapy] at the *Centro Studi in Psicoterapia Cognitiva Costruttivista* [Center for Studies in Cognitive Constructivist Psychotherapy]: https://www.cesipc.it
- Short specialization program: Personal Construct Psychology and Counseling (PC2; University of Padua): https://uel.unipd.it/en/masters/pc2-personal-construct-psychology-and-counselling/
- The Taos Institute: https://www.taosinstitute.net/education/workshops-courses/introduction-to-social-construction
- Vancouver School for Narrative Therapy: https://www.vancouverschoolfornarrativetherapy.com/

References

Ainsworth, C., & Nature Magazine. (2018, October 22). Sex redefined: The idea of 2 sexes is overly simplistic. *Scientific American.* https://www.scientificamerican.com/article/sex-redefined-the-idea-of-2-sexes-is-overly-simplistic1/

Alesina, A., Giuliano, P., & Nunn, N. (2013). On the origins of gender roles: Women and the plough. *The Quarterly Journal of Economics, 128*(2), 469–530. https://doi.org/10.1093/qje/qjt005

Alexander, F., & French, T. M. (1946). *Psychoanalytic therapy: Principles and applications.* Ronald Press.

Alexander, P. C., Neimeyer, R. A., & Follette, V. M. (1991). Group therapy for women sexually abused as children: A controlled study and investigation of individual differences. *Journal of Interpersonal Violence, 6*(2), 218–231. https://doi.org/10.1177/088626091006002006

Alexander, P. C., Neimeyer, R. A., Follette, V. M., Moore, M. K., & Harter, S. (1989). A comparison of group treatments of women sexually abused as children. *Journal of Consulting and Clinical Psychology, 57*(4), 479–483. https://doi.org/10.1037/0022-006X.57.4.479

Alves, D., Mendes, I., Gonçalves, M. M., & Neimeyer, R. A. (2012). Innovative moments in grief therapy: Reconstructing meaning following perinatal death. *Death Studies, 36*(9), 795–818. https://doi.org/10.1080/07481187.2011.608291

American Psychiatric Association. (2022). *Diagnostic and statistical manual of mental disorders* (5th ed., text rev.). https://doi.org/10.1176/appi.books.9780890425787

American Psychological Association. (2017). *Multicultural guidelines: An ecological approach to context, identity, and intersectionality.* https://doi.org/10.1037/e501962018-001

REFERENCES

Bannister, D., Adams-Webber, J. R., Penn, W. I., & Radley, A. R. (1975). Reversing the process of thought disorder: A serial validation experiment. *The British Journal of Social and Clinical Psychology*, *14*(2), 169–180. https://doi.org/10.1111/j.2044-8260.1975.tb00165.x

Batista, J., Silva, J., Freitas, S., Alves, D., Machado, A., Sousa, I., Fernández-Navarro, P., Magalhães, C., & Gonçalves, M. M. (2019). Relational schemas as mediators of innovative moments in symptom improvement in major depression. *Psychotherapy Research*, *29*(1), 58–69. https://doi.org/10.1080/10503307.2017.1359427

Batista, J., Silva, J., Magalhães, C., Ferreira, H., Fernández-Navarro, P., & Gonçalves, M. M. (2020). Studying psychotherapy change in narrative terms: The innovative moments method. *Counselling & Psychotherapy Research*, *20*(3), 442–448. https://doi.org/10.1002/capr.12297

Beail, N., & Parker, S. (1991). Group fixed-role therapy: A clinical application. *International Journal of Personal Construct Psychology*, *4*(1), 85–95. https://doi.org/10.1080/08936039108404762

Beaudoin, M.-N., Moersch, M., & Evare, B. S. (2016). The effectiveness of narrative therapy with children's social and emotional skill development: An empirical study of 813 problem-solving stories. *Journal of Systemic Therapies*, *35*(3), 42–59. https://doi.org/10.1521/jsyt.2016.35.3.42

Beaudoin, M.-N., Tan, A., Gannon, C., & Moersch, M. (2017). A comparative study of the effects of 6, 12, and 16 weeks of narrative therapy on social and emotional skills: An empirical analysis of 722 children's problem-solving accounts. *Journal of Systemic Therapies*, *36*(4), 57–73. https://doi.org/10.1521/jsyt.2017.36.4.57

Beck, A. T. (2019). A 60-year evolution of cognitive theory and therapy. *Perspectives on Psychological Science*, *14*(1), 16–20. https://doi.org/10.1177/1745691618804187

Beck, A. T., Rush, A. J., Shaw, B. F., & Emery, G. (1979). *Cognitive therapy of depression*. The Guilford Press.

Berkeley, G. (2009). *A treatise concerning the principles of human knowledge*. Project Gutenberg. https://www.gutenberg.org/files/4723/4723-h/4723-h.htm (Original work published 1710)

Berry, F. M. (1984). An introduction to Stephen C. Pepper's philosophical system via World Hypotheses: A Study in Evidence. *Bulletin of the Psychonomic Society*, *22*(5), 446–448. https://doi.org/10.3758/BF03333873

Bertalanffy, L. von. (1972). The history and status of general systems theory. *Academy of Management Journal*, *15*(4), 407–426. https://doi.org/10.2307/255139 (Reprinted from *Trends in general systems theory*, pp. 21–41, by G. J. Klir, Ed., 1972, Wiley-Interscience)

REFERENCES

Bohart, A. C., O'Hara, M., & Leitner, L. M. (1998). Empirically violated treatments: Disenfranchisement of humanistic and other psychotherapies. *Psychotherapy Research, 8*(2), 141–157. https://doi.org/10.1080/10503309812331332277

Bonarius, J. C. (1970). Fixed role therapy: A double paradox. *The British Journal of Medical Psychology, 43*(3), 213–219. https://doi.org/10.1111/j.2044-8341.1970.tb02119.x

Bonazzi, M. (2020). Protagoras. In E. N. Zalta (Ed.), *The Stanford encyclopedia of philosophy archive* (Fall 2020 ed.). Stanford University. https://plato.stanford.edu/archives/fall2020/entries/protagoras/

Botella, L. (2000). PCP, constructivism, and psychotherapy research. In J. W. Scheer (Ed.), *The person in society: Challenges to a constructivist theory* (pp. 362–372). Psychosozial-Verlag.

Bowen, M. (1978). *Family therapy in clinical practice*. Jason Aronson.

Bridges, S. K., & Raskin, J. D. (in press). A brief introduction to constructivist psychotherapy. In L. Hoffman (Ed.), *APA handbook of humanistic and existential psychology: Vol. 2. Clinical and social applications*. American Psychological Association.

Brown, L. S. (2000). Discomforts of the powerless: Feminist constructions of distress. In R. A. Neimeyer & J. D. Raskin (Eds.), *Constructions of disorder: Meaning-making frameworks for psychotherapy* (pp. 287–308). American Psychological Association. https://doi.org/10.1037/10368-012

Brown, L. S. (2018). *Feminist therapy* (2nd ed.). American Psychological Association. https://doi.org/10.1037/0000092-000

Brown, R., & Chiesa, M. (1990). An introduction to repertory grid theory and technique. *British Journal of Psychotherapy, 6*(4), 411–419. https://doi.org/10.1111/j.1752-0118.1990.tb01302.x

Burr, V. (2025). *Social constructionism* (4th ed.). Routledge. https://doi.org/10.4324/9781003335016

Butt, T. (2000). Pragmatism, constructivism, and ethics. *Journal of Constructivist Psychology, 13*(2), 85–101. https://doi.org/10.1080/107205300265892

Butt, T., & Parton, N. (2005). Constructive social work and personal construct theory: The case of psychological trauma. *British Journal of Social Work, 35*(6), 793–806. https://doi.org/10.1093/bjsw/bch210

Button, E. J. (1987). Construing people or weight?: An eating disorders group. In R. A. Neimeyer & G. J. Neimeyer (Eds.), *Personal construct therapy casebook* (pp. 230–244). Springer Publishing Company.

Cahn, L. (2024, October 1). How pink and blue became the "girl" and "boy" baby colors. *Reader's Digest*. https://www.rd.com/article/pink-for-boys/

Cain, D. J. (2010). *Person-centered psychotherapies*. American Psychological Association. https://doi.org/10.1037/17330-000

Cambridge University Press & Assessment. (n.d.). Philology. In *Cambridge dictionary*. Retrieved July 8, 2024, from https://dictionary.cambridge.org/us/dictionary/english/philology

Cameron, J. (2020, August 31). Why red means stop and green means go: Getting There. *CT Post*. https://www.ctpost.com/news/article/Why-red-means-stop-and-green-means-go-Getting-15525851.php

Casey, P. (2016, July 25). Patient, service user or client-what's in a name? *Irish Independent*. https://www.independent.ie/life/health-wellbeing/healthy-eating/patient-service-user-or-client-whats-in-a-name/34904915.html

Cashdan, S. (1988). *Object relations therapy: Using the relationship*. W. W. Norton & Company.

Cashin, A., Browne, G., Bradbury, J., & Mulder, A. (2013). The effectiveness of narrative therapy with young people with autism. *Journal of Child and Adolescent Psychiatric Nursing, 26*(1), 32–41. https://doi.org/10.1111/jcap.12020

Clapton, E. (1986). It's in the way that you use it [Song]. On *August*. Duck Records/Warner Bros. Records.

Cobern, W. W., & Loving, C. C. (2008). An essay for educators: Epistemological realism really is common sense. *Science & Education, 17*(4), 425–447. https://doi.org/10.1007/s11191-007-9095-5

Conti, J., Heywood, L., Hay, P., Shrestha, R. M., & Perich, T. (2022). Paper 2: A systematic review of narrative therapy treatment outcomes for eating disorders—Bridging the divide between practice-based evidence and evidence-based practice. *Journal of Eating Disorders, 10*, Article 138. https://doi.org/10.1186/s40337-022-00636-4

Costa, D. S. J., Mercieca-Bebber, R., Tesson, S., Seidler, Z., & Lopez, A.-L. (2019). Patient, client, consumer, survivor or other alternatives? A scoping review of preferred terms for labelling individuals who access healthcare across settings. *BMJ Open, 9*(3), Article e025166. https://doi.org/10.1136/bmjopen-2018-025166

Cromwell, R. L. (2010). *Being human: Human being. A manifesto for a new psychology*. iUniverse.

Cunha, C. A. C., Spínola, J., & Gonçalves, M. M. (2012). The emergence of innovative moments in narrative therapy for depression: Exploring therapist and client contributions. *Research in Psychotherapy: Psychopathology, Process and Outcome, 15*(2), 62–74. https://doi.org/10.4081/ripppo.2012.120

Curtis, R. C., & Hirsch, I. (2003). Relational approaches to psychoanalytic psychotherapy. In A. S. Gurman & S. B. Messer (Eds.), *Essential psychotherapies: Theory and practice* (2nd ed., pp. 69–106). The Guilford Press.

Cutolo, M. (2023, July 12). This is why traffic lights are red, yellow and green. *Reader's Digest*. https://www.rd.com/article/traffic-lights/

REFERENCES

Dobson, K. S. (2001). *Handbook of cognitive–behavioral therapies* (2nd ed.). The Guilford Press.

Doherty, W. J., & McDaniel, S. H. (2009). *Family therapy*. American Psychological Association. https://doi.org/10.1037/12062-000

Domenici, V. A. (2007). *Experiential personal construct psychology and depression: A qualitative study* [Doctoral dissertation, Miami University]. OhioLINK. https://etd.ohiolink.edu/acprod/odb_etd/etd/r/1501/10?clear=10&p10_accession_num=miami1195061434

Drüge, M., Staeck, R., Haller, E., Seiler, C., Rohner, V., & Watzke, B. (2023). Innovative moments in low-intensity, telephone-based cognitive-behavioral therapy for depression. *Frontiers in Psychology, 14*, Article 1165899. https://doi.org/10.3389/fpsyg.2023.1165899

Ecker, B. (2020). Erasing problematic emotional learnings. In R. D. Lane & L. Nadel (Eds.), *Neuroscience of enduring change: Implications for psychotherapy* (pp. 273–299). Oxford University Press. https://doi.org/10.1093/oso/9780190881511.003.0011

Ecker, B., & Bridges, S. K. (2020). How the science of memory reconsolidation advances the effectiveness and unification of psychotherapy. *Clinical Social Work Journal, 48*(3), 287–300. https://doi.org/10.1007/s10615-020-00754-z

Ecker, B., & Hulley, L. (1996). *Depth-oriented brief therapy*. Jossey-Bass Publishers.

Ecker, B., & Hulley, L. (2008). Coherence therapy: Swift change at the core of emotional truth. In J. D. Raskin & S. K. Bridges (Eds.), *Studies in meaning 3: Constructivist psychotherapy in the real world* (pp. 57–84). Pace University Press.

Efran, J. (2020, January/February). In search of new ideas: My evolution as a therapist. *Psychotherapy Networker*. https://www.psychotherapynetworker.org/article/search-new-ideas/

Efran, J., & Fauber, R. (2015, March/April). Spitting in the client's soup: Don't overthink your interventions. *Psychotherapy Networker*. https://www.psychotherapynetworker.org/article/spitting-clients-soup/

Efran, J., Lukens, M., & Lukens, M. (2007, March/April). Defining psychotherapy: The last 25 years have taught us that it's neither art nor science. *Psychotherapy Networker*. https://www.psychotherapynetworker.org/article/defining-psychotherapy/

Efran, J. S. (2022). Upsetting apple carts. *Cybernetics & Human Knowing, 29*(1–2), 25–34.

Efran, J. S. (2024, May/June). Experiments in being someone else. *Psychotherapy Networker*, 50–53. https://www.psychotherapynetworker.org/article/experiments-in-being-someone-else/

Efran, J. S., & Fauber, R. L. (1995). Radical constructivism: Questions and answers. In R. A. Neimeyer & M. J. Mahoney (Eds.), *Constructivism in psychotherapy* (pp. 275–304). American Psychological Association. https://doi.org/10.1037/10170-012

Efran, J. S., & Heffner, K. P. (1998). Is constructivist psychotherapy epistemologically flawed? *Journal of Constructivist Psychology*, *11*(2), 89–103. https://doi.org/10.1080/10720539808404642

Efran, J. S., Lukens, M. D., & Lukens, R. J. (1990). *Language, structure, and change: Frameworks of meaning in psychotherapy.* W. W. Norton & Co.

Efran, J. S., McNamee, S., Warren, B., & Raskin, J. D. (2014). Personal construct psychology, radical constructivism, and social constructionism: A dialogue. *Journal of Constructivist Psychology*, *27*(1), 1–13. https://doi.org/10.1080/10720537.2014.850367

Efran, J. S., & Nath, S. R. (2004). The Zen of social phobia: A context-centered group treatment. In J. D. Raskin & S. K. Bridges (Eds.), *Studies in meaning 2: Bridging the personal and social in constructivist psychology* (pp. 185–219). Pace University Press.

Efran, J. S., & Sitrin, L. C. (2002). Context-centered therapy. In R. A. DiTomasso & E. A. Gosch (Eds.), *Anxiety disorders: A practitioner's guide to comparative treatments* (pp. 137–159). Springer Publishing.

Efran, J. S., & Soler-Baillo, J. (2008). Mind and self in context-centered psychotherapy. In J. D. Raskin & S. K. Bridges (Eds.), *Studies in meaning 3: Constructivist psychotherapy in the real world* (pp. 85–105). Pace University Press.

Einstein, A., & Infeld, L. (1938). *The evolution of physics.* The Scientific Book Club. https://archive.org/details/evolutionofphysi033254mbp/page/n7/mode/2up

Ellis, A. (1997). Postmodern ethics for active-directive counseling and psychotherapy. *Journal of Mental Health Counseling*, *19*(3), 211–225.

Ellis, A. (1998). How rational emotive behavior therapy belongs in the constructivist camp. In M. F. Hoyt (Ed.), *The handbook of constructive therapies: Innovative approaches from leading practitioners* (pp. 83–99). Jossey-Bass/Wiley.

Ellis, A., & Joffe Ellis, D. (2019). *Rational emotive behavior therapy* (2nd ed.). American Psychological Association. https://doi.org/10.1037/0000134-000

Epting, F. R. (1984). *Personal construct counseling and psychotherapy.* John Wiley & Sons.

Epting, F. R., & Leitner, L. M. (1992). Humanistic psychology and personal construct theory. *The Humanistic Psychologist*, *20*(2–3), 243–259. https://doi.org/10.1080/08873267.1992.9986793

Epting, F. R., & Nazario, A., Jr. (1987). Designing a fixed role therapy: Issues, techniques, and modifications. In R. A. Neimeyer & G. J. Neimeyer (Eds.), *Personal construct therapy casebook* (pp. 277–289). Springer Publishing Company.

REFERENCES

Epting, F. R., & Paris, M. E. (2006). A constructive understanding of the person: George Kelly and humanistic psychology. *The Humanistic Psychologist*, *34*(1), 21–37. https://doi.org/10.1207/s15473333thp3401_4

Eron, J. B., & Lund, T. W. (1993). How problems evolve and dissolve: Integrating narrative and strategic concepts. *Family Process*, *32*(3), 291–309. https://doi.org/10.1111/j.1545-5300.1993.00291.x

Eron, J. B., & Lund, T. W. (1996). *Narrative solutions in brief therapy*. The Guilford Press.

Eron, J. B., & Lund, T. W. (2002). Narrative solutions: Toward understanding the art of helpful conversation. In J. D. Raskin & S. K. Bridges (Eds.), *Studies in meaning: Exploring constructivist psychology* (pp. 63–97). Pace University Press.

Esfahani, M., Kajbaf, M., & Abedi, M. (2015). Evaluation and comparison of the effects of time perspective therapy, acceptance and commitment therapy and narrative therapy on severity of symptoms of obsessive-compulsive disorder. *Journal of the Indian Academy of Applied Psychology*, *41*(3), 149–156.

Esposito, G., Cutolo, A. S., Passeggia, R., Formentin, S., & Gonçalves, M. M. (2022). Tracking change in group interventions: A further adaptation of the innovative moments coding system for groups. *Research in Psychotherapy*, *25*(3), 354–364. https://doi.org/10.4081/ripppo.2022.648

Esposito, G., Cutolo, A. S., Passeggia, R., Oliveira, J. T., & Gonçalves, M. M. (2024). Reliability of the innovative moments coding system for groups and the association between markers of change and outcomes. *Group Dynamics*, *28*(2), 82–100. https://doi.org/10.1037/gdn0000212

Esposito, G., Passeggia, R., Cutolo, A. S., Karterud, S., & Freda, M. F. (2020). Treatment integrity and members' change in group counseling: A pilot study on counselor's mentalizing interventions. *Professional Psychology, Research and Practice*, *51*(6), 588–597. https://doi.org/10.1037/pro0000304

Faidley, A. F., & Leitner, L. M. (1993). *Assessing experience in psychotherapy: Personal construct alternatives*. Praeger Publishers/Greenwood Publishing Group.

Fallah, K., & Ghodsi, M. (2022). The effectiveness of narrative therapy on sexual function and couple burnout. *Revista Portuguesa de Investigação Comportamental e Social*, *8*(1), 1–13. https://doi.org/10.31211//rpics.2022.8.1.219

Faulkenberry, E. D., & Faulkenberry, T. J. (2006, April). Constructivism in mathematics education: A historical and personal perspective. *The Texas Science Teacher*, 17–21.

Feixas, G., Bados, A., García-Grau, E., Paz, C., Montesano, A., Compañ, V., Salla, M., Aguilera, M., Trujillo, A., Cañete, J., Medeiros-Ferreira, L., Soriano, J.,

Ibarra, M., Medina, J. C., Ortíz, E., & Lana, F. (2016). A dilemma-focused intervention for depression: A multicenter, randomized controlled trial with a 3-month follow-up. *Depression and Anxiety, 33*(9), 862–869. https://doi.org/10.1002/da.22510

Feixas, G., & Compañ, V. (2016). Dilemma-focused intervention for unipolar depression: A treatment manual. *BMC Psychiatry, 16*, Article 235. https://doi.org/10.1186/s12888-016-0947-x

Fernández-Navarro, P., Ribeiro, A. P., Soylemez, K. K., & Gonçalves, M. M. (2020). Innovative moments as developmental change levels: A case study on meaning integration in the treatment of depression. *Journal of Constructivist Psychology, 33*(2), 207–223. https://doi.org/10.1080/10720537.2019.1592037

Fernández-Navarro, P., Rosa, C., Sousa, I., Moutinho, V., Antunes, A., Magalhães, C., Ribeiro, A. P., & Gonçalves, M. M. (2018). Reconceptualization innovative moments as a predictor of symptomatology improvement in treatment for depression. *Clinical Psychology & Psychotherapy, 25*(6), 765–773. https://doi.org/10.1002/cpp.2306

Fowers, B. J. (2010). Instrumentalism and psychology: Beyond using and being used. *Theory & Psychology, 20*(1), 102–124. https://doi.org/10.1177/0959354309346080

Fox, A. (2020, June 18). Compared with hummingbirds, people are rather colorblind. *Smithsonian Magazine.* https://www.smithsonianmag.com/smart-news/compared-hummingbirds-were-all-colorblind-180975111/

Frank, J. D., & Frank, J. B. (1991). *Persuasion and healing: A comparative study of psychotherapy* (3rd ed.). The Johns Hopkins University Press.

Freeman, A., Mahoney, M. J., DeVito, P., & Martin, D. (Eds.). (2004). *Cognition and psychotherapy.* Springer Publishing Company.

Freud, S. (1960). *The ego and the id* (J. Riviere Trans.; J. Strachey, Ed.). W. W. Norton and Company. (Original work published 1923)

Freud, S. (1965). *New introductory lectures on psychoanalysis* (J. Strachey, Trans.). W. W. Norton and Company. (Original work published 1933)

Fromm, M. (2004). *Introduction to the repertory grid interview.* Waxmann Münster.

Garcia-Martínez, J., Maestre-Castillo, D., Payán-Bravo, M. A., & Fernández-Navarro, P. (2021). Innovative moments in group therapy: Analyzing voices of group change. *Journal of Constructivist Psychology, 34*(2), 195–206. https://doi.org/10.1080/10720537.2020.1717143

Gash, H., & Glasersfeld, E. von. (1978). Vico (1668–2744): An early anticipator of radical constructivism. *The Irish Journal of Psychology, 4*(1), 22–32. https://doi.org/10.1080/03033910.1978.10557633

Gergen, K. J. (1994). *Realities and relationships: Soundings in social construction.* Harvard University Press.

Gergen, K. J. (1995). Postmodernism as a humanism. *The Humanistic Psychologist, 23*(1), 71–82. https://doi.org/10.1080/08873267.1995.9986816

Gergen, K. J. (2015). *An invitation to social construction* (3rd ed.). SAGE Publications. https://doi.org/10.4135/9781473921276

Ghavibazou, E., Hosseinian, S., Ghamari Kivi, H., & Ale Ebrahim, N. (2022). Narrative therapy, applications, and outcomes: A systematic review. *Preventive Counseling, 2*(4), 1–11. https://jpc.uma.ac.ir/article_1596.html

Glasersfeld, E. von. (1984). An introduction to radical constructivism. In P. Watzlawick (Ed.), *The invented reality: How do we know what we believe we know? Contributions to constructivism* (pp. 17–40). W. W. Norton & Company.

Glasersfeld, E. von. (1995). *Radical constructivism: A way of knowing and learning.* The Falmer Press.

Glasersfeld, E. von. (2007). Aspects of constructivism: Vico, Berkeley, Piaget. In M. Larochelle (Ed.), *Key works in radical constructivism* (pp. 91–99). Sense Publishers. (Original work published 1992)

Gonçalves, M. M., Batista, J., Braga, C., Oliveira, J. T., Fernandéz-Navarro, P., Magalhães, C., Ferreira, H., & Sousa, I. (2022). Innovative moments in recovered cases treated with the unified protocol for transdiagnostic treatment of emotional disorders. *Psychotherapy Research, 32*(6), 736–747. https://doi.org/10.1080/10503307.2021.2003463

Gonçalves, M. M., Matos, M., & Santos, A. (2009). Narrative therapy and the nature of "innovative moments" in the construction of change. *Journal of Constructivist Psychology, 22*(1), 1–23. https://doi.org/10.1080/10720530802500748

Gonçalves, M. M., Ribeiro, A. P., Mendes, I., Matos, M., & Santos, A. (2011). Tracking novelties in psychotherapy process research: The innovative moments coding system. *Psychotherapy Research, 21*(5), 497–509. https://doi.org/10.1080/10503307.2011.560207

Gonçalves, M. M., Ribeiro, A. P., Silva, J. R., Mendes, I., & Sousa, I. (2016). Narrative innovations predict symptom improvement: Studying innovative moments in narrative therapy of depression. *Psychotherapy Research, 26*(4), 425–435. https://doi.org/10.1080/10503307.2015.1035355

Google. (n.d.). Constructive. In *Google dictionary*. Retrieved July 13, 2024, from https://g.co/kgs/Q9FuECm

Graham, D. W. (2019). Heraclitus. In E. N. Zalta (Ed.), *The Stanford encyclopedia of philosophy archive* (Summer 2021 ed.). Stanford University. https://plato.stanford.edu/archives/sum2021/entries/heraclitus/

Hawke, L. D., Nguyen, A. T. P., Rodak, T., Yanos, P. T., & Castle, D. J. (2023). Narrative-based psychotherapies for mood disorders: A scoping review of the literature. *SSM—Mental Health, 3*, Article 137. https://doi.org/10.1016/j.ssmmh.2023.100224

REFERENCES

Hayes, S. C., Follette, V. M., & Linehan, M. M. (Eds.). (2004). *Mindfulness and acceptance: Expanding the cognitive-behavioral tradition.* The Guilford Press.

Held, B. S. (1995). *Back to reality: A critique of postmodern theory in psychotherapy.* W. W. Norton & Company.

Held, B. S. (1998). The many truths of postmodernist discourse. *Journal of Theoretical and Philosophical Psychology, 18*(2), 193–217. https://doi.org/10.1037/h0091185

Heywood, L., Conti, J., & Hay, P. (2022). Paper 1: A systematic synthesis of narrative therapy treatment components for the treatment of eating disorders. *Journal of Eating Disorders, 10,* Article 137. https://doi.org/10.1186/s40337-022-00635-5

Higgins, C. F. (n.d.). Gorgias. In J. Fieser & B. Dowden (Eds.), *Internet encyclopedia of philosophy.* Retrieved July 8, 2024, from https://iep.utm.edu/gorgias/

Hinkle, D. N. (1965). *The change of personal constructs from the viewpoint of a theory of construct implications* [Doctoral dissertation, The Ohio State University]. http://www.pcp-net.org/journal/pctp10/hinkle1965.pdf

Holland, J. M., & Neimeyer, R. A. (2009). The efficacy of personal construct therapy as a function of the type and severity of the presenting problem. *Journal of Constructivist Psychology, 22*(2), 170–185. https://doi.org/10.1080/10720530802675904

Holland, J. M., Neimeyer, R. A., Currier, J. M., & Berman, J. S. (2007). The efficacy of personal construct therapy: A comprehensive review. *Journal of Clinical Psychology, 63*(1), 93–107. https://doi.org/10.1002/jclp.20332

Holland, R. (1970). George Kelly: Constructive innocent and reluctant existentialist. In D. Bannister (Ed.), *Perspectives in personal construct theory* (pp. 111–132). Academic Press.

Horley, J. (2005). Fixed-role therapy with multiple paraphilias. *Clinical Case Studies, 4*(1), 72–80. https://doi.org/10.1177/1534650103259675

Horley, J. (2006). Personal construct psychotherapy: Fixed-role therapy with forensic clients. *Journal of Sexual Aggression, 12*(1), 53–61. https://doi.org/10.1080/13552600600673596

Hoyt, M. F. (Ed.). (1994). *Constructive therapies* (Vol. 1). The Guilford Press.

Hoyt, M. F. (Ed.). (1996). *Constructive therapies* (Vol. 2). The Guilford Press.

Hume, D. (2006). *An enquiry concerning human understanding* (L. A. Selby-Bigge, Ed.). Project Gutenberg. https://www.gutenberg.org/ebooks/9662 (Original work published 1777)

Hussey, K. A., Hadyniak, S. E., & Johnston, R. J., Jr. (2022). Patterning and development of photoreceptors in the human retina. *Frontiers in Cell and Developmental Biology, 10,* Article 878350. https://doi.org/10.3389/fcell.2022.878350

Iglesias, A., & Iglesias, A. (2014). Hypnosis aided fixed role therapy for social phobia: A case report. *The American Journal of Clinical Hypnosis, 56*(4), 405–412. https://doi.org/10.1080/00029157.2013.808166

Ikonomopoulos, J., Smith, R. L., & Schmidt, C. (2015). Integrating narrative therapy within rehabilitative programming for incarcerated adolescents. *Journal of Counseling and Development, 93*(4), 460–470. https://doi.org/10.1002/jcad.12044

Jalali, F., Hashemi, S. F., & Hasani, A. (2019). Narrative therapy for depression and anxiety among children with imprisoned parents: A randomised pilot efficacy trial. *Journal of Child and Adolescent Mental Health, 31*(3), 189–200. https://doi.org/10.2989/17280583.2019.1678474

Jankowicz, D. (2003). *The easy guide to repertory grids.* Wiley.

Juvova, A., Chudy, S., Neumeister, P., Plischke, J., & Kvintova, J. (2015). Reflection of constructivist theories in current educational practice. *Universal Journal of Educational Research, 3*(5), 345–349. https://doi.org/10.13189/ujer.2015.030506

Kamens, S. R., Elkins, D. N., & Robbins, B. D. (2017). Open letter to the DSM-5. *Journal of Humanistic Psychology, 57*(6), 675–687. https://doi.org/10.1177/0022167817698261

Kant, I. (1990). *Critique of pure reason* (J. M. D. Meiklejohn, Trans.). Prometheus Books. (Original work published 1781)

Kant, I. (2004). *Prolegomena to any future metaphysics: With selections from the Critique of Pure Reason* (G. Hatfield, Ed. & Trans.; rev. ed.). Cambridge University Press. https://doi.org/10.1017/CBO9780511808517 (Original work published 1783)

Karibwende, F., Niyonsenga, J., Nyirinkwaya, S., Hitayezu, I., Sebuhoro, C., Simeon Sebatukura, G. S., Marie Ntete, J. M., & Mutabaruka, J. (2022). A randomized controlled trial evaluating the effectiveness of narrative therapy on resilience of orphaned and abandoned children fostered in SOS children's village. *European Journal of Psychotraumatology, 13*(2), Article 215211. https://doi.org/10.1080/20008066.2022.2152111

Kelly, G. A. (1955a). *The psychology of personal constructs: Vol. 1. A theory of personality.* W. W. Norton.

Kelly, G. A. (1955b). *The psychology of personal constructs: Vol. 2. Clinical diagnosis and psychotherapy.* W. W. Norton.

Kelly, G. A. (1966, April). *Behavior is a question* [Undelivered paper due to illness]. 10th Inter-American Congress of Psychology, Lima, Peru. Fransella PCP Collection, University of Hertfordshire, University Library Archives.

REFERENCES

Kelly, G. A. (1967). *Personal construct theory bibliography supplement* [Unpublished manuscript]. Fransella PCP Collection, University of Hertfordshire, University Library Archives.

Kelly, G. A. (1969a). The autobiography of a theory. In B. Maher (Ed.), *Clinical psychology and personality: The selected papers of George Kelly* (pp. 46–65). John Wiley & Sons. (Previously unpublished work written in 1963)

Kelly, G. A. (1969b). The language of hypothesis: Man's psychological instrument. In B. Maher (Ed.), *Clinical psychology and personality: The selected papers of George Kelly* (pp. 147–162). John Wiley & Sons. (Reprinted from "The language of hypothesis: Man's psychological instrument," 1964, *Journal of Individual Psychology, 20*[2], 137–152)

Kelly, G. A. (1969c). Man's construction of his alternatives. In B. Maher (Ed.), *Clinical psychology and personality: The selected papers of George Kelly* (pp. 66–93). John Wiley & Sons. (Reprinted from *Assessment of human motives*, pp. 33–64, by G. Lindzey, Ed., 1958, Holt, Rinehart & Winston)

Kelly, G. A. (1969d). Ontological acceleration. In B. Maher (Ed.), *Clinical psychology and personality: The selected papers of George Kelly* (pp. 7–45). John Wiley & Sons. (Previously unpublished work written in 1966)

Kelly, G. A. (1969e). Personal construct theory and the psychotherapeutic interview. In B. Maher (Ed.), *Clinical psychology and personality: The selected papers of George Kelly* (pp. 224–264). John Wiley & Sons. (Previously unpublished work written in 1958)

Kelly, G. A. (1970). Behaviour is an experiment. In D. Bannister (Ed.), *Perspectives in personal construct theory* (pp. 255–269). Academic Press. (Previously unpublished work written in 1966)

Kelly, G. A. (1973). Fixed role therapy. In R.-R. M. Jerjevich (Ed.), *Direct psychotherapy: 28 American originals* (Vol. 1, pp. 394–422). University of Miami Press. https://doi.org/10.4324/9780203405970

Kelly, G. A. (1977). The psychology of the unknown. In D. Bannister (Ed.), *New perspectives in personal construct theory* (pp. 1–19). Academic Press.

Korzybski, A. (1994). *Science and sanity: An introduction to non-Aristotelian systems and general semantics* (5th ed.). Institute of General Semantics.

Koutoufa, I., Conceição, E., Sousa, I., Evangeli, M., Crosby, R., Wonderlich, S., & Mendes, I. (2024). Innovative moments and the process of change in the treatment of bulimia nervosa. *Journal of Constructivist Psychology, 37*(1), 62–76. https://doi.org/10.1080/10720537.2023.2235706

Landfield, A. W. (1971). *Personal construct systems in psychotherapy*. Rand McNally.

Lane, L. G., & Viney, L. L. (2005). The effects of personal construct group therapy on breast cancer survivors. *Journal of Consulting and Clinical Psychology, 73*(2), 284–292. https://doi.org/10.1037/0022-006X.73.2.284

REFERENCES

Lane, L. G., & Viney, L. L. (2006). When the unreal becomes real: An evaluation of personal construct group psychotherapy with survivors of breast cancer. In P. Caputi, H. Foster, & L. L. Viney (Eds.), *Personal construct psychology: New ideas* (pp. 241-251). John Wiley & Sons. https://doi.org/10.1002/9780470713044.ch19

Langer, E. (1989). *Mindfulness*. Addison-Wesley.

Leitner, L., & Thomas, J. (2003). Experiential personal construct psychotherapy. In F. Fransella (Ed.), *International handbook of personal construct psychology* (pp. 257-264). John Wiley & Sons. https://doi.org/10.1002/0470013370.ch25

Leitner, L. M. (1988). Terror, risk, and reverence: Experiential personal construct psychotherapy. *International Journal of Personal Construct Psychology, 1*(3), 251-261. https://doi.org/10.1080/10720538808409398

Leitner, L. M. (1995). Optimal therapeutic distance: A therapist's experience of personal construct psychotherapy. In R. A. Neimeyer & M. J. Mahoney (Eds.), *Constructivism in psychotherapy* (pp. 357-370). American Psychological Association. https://doi.org/10.1037/10170-015

Leitner, L. M. (1999). Levels of awareness in experiential personal construct psychotherapy. *Journal of Constructivist Psychology, 12*(3), 239-252. https://doi.org/10.1080/107205399266091

Leitner, L. M., & Faidley, A. F. (2002). Disorder, diagnoses, and the struggles of humanness. In J. D. Raskin & S. K. Bridges (Eds.), *Studies in meaning: Exploring constructivist psychology* (pp. 99-121). Pace University Press.

Leitner, L. M., & Faidley, A. J. (1999). Creativity in experiential personal construct psychotherapy. *Journal of Constructivist Psychology, 12*(4), 273-286. https://doi.org/10.1080/107205399266019

Lesher, J. H. (1978). Xenophanes' scepticism. *Phronesis, 23*(1), 1-21. https://doi.org/10.1163/156852878X00181

Levenson, H. (2017). *Brief dynamic therapy* (2nd ed.). American Psychological Association. https://doi.org/10.1037/0000043-000

Lira, F. T., Nay, W. R., McCullough, J. P., & Etkin, M. W. (1975). Relative effects of modeling and role playing in the treatment of avoidance behaviors. *Journal of Consulting and Clinical Psychology, 43*(5), 608-618. https://doi.org/10.1037/0022-006X.43.5.608

Locke, J. (2019). *An essay concerning human understanding*. Global Grey. https://www.globalgreyebooks.com/essay-concerning-human-understanding-ebook.html (Original work published 1690)

Looyeh, M. Y., Kamali, K., Ghasemi, A., & Tonawanik, P. (2014). Treating social phobia in children through group narrative therapy. *The Arts in Psychotherapy, 41*(1), 16-20. https://doi.org/10.1016/j.aip.2013.11.005

Looyeh, M. Y., Kamali, K., & Shafieian, R. (2012). An exploratory study of the effectiveness of group narrative therapy on the school behavior of girls with attention-deficit/hyperactivity symptoms. *Archives of Psychiatric Nursing, 26*(5), 404–410. https://doi.org/10.1016/j.apnu.2012.01.001

Lopes, R. T., Gonçalves, M. M., Fassnacht, D. B., Machado, P. P. P., & Sousa, I. (2014). Long-term effects of psychotherapy on moderate depression: A comparative study of narrative therapy and cognitive-behavioral therapy. *Journal of Affective Disorders, 167*, 64–73. https://doi.org/10.1016/j.jad.2014.05.042

Lopes, R. T., Gonçalves, M. M., Machado, P. P. P., Sinai, D., Bento, T., & Salgado, J. (2014). Narrative therapy vs. cognitive-behavioral therapy for moderate depression: Empirical evidence from a controlled clinical trial. *Psychotherapy Research, 24*(6), 662–674. https://doi.org/10.1080/10503307.2013.874052

Lyddon, W. J. (1989). Root metaphor theory: A philosophical framework for counseling and psychotherapy. *Journal of Counseling and Development, 67*(8), 442–448. https://doi.org/10.1002/j.1556-6676.1989.tb02113.x

Lyddon, W. J. (1995). Forms and facets of constructivist psychology. In R. A. Neimeyer & M. J. Mahoney (Eds.), *Constructivism in psychotherapy* (pp. 69–92). American Psychological Association. https://doi.org/10.1037/10170-003

Lynch, F. L., Dickerson, J. F., Rozenman, M. S., Gonzalez, A., Schwartz, K. T. G., Porta, G., O'Keeffe-Rosetti, M., Brent, D., & Weersing, V. R. (2021). Cost-effectiveness of brief behavioral therapy for pediatric anxiety and depression in primary care. *JAMA Network Open, 4*(3), Article e211778. https://doi.org/10.1001/jamanetworkopen.2021.1778

Mackay, N. (2003). Psychotherapy and the idea of meaning. *Theory & Psychology, 13*(3), 359–386. https://doi.org/10.1177/0959354303013003004

Mackay, N. (2011). On some accounts of meaning and their problems. In N. Mackay & A. Petocz (Eds.), *Realism and psychology: Collected essays* (pp. 548–596). Brill. https://doi.org/10.1163/9789004194878_017

Madigan, S. (2025). *Narrative therapy* (3rd ed.). American Psychological Association.

Mahoney, M. J. (1988). Constructive metatheory: I. Basic features and historical foundations. *International Journal of Personal Construct Psychology, 1*(1), 1–35. https://doi.org/10.1080/10720538808412762

Mahoney, M. J. (1991). *Human change processes*. Basic Books.

Mahoney, M. J. (2003). *Constructive psychotherapy: A practical guide*. The Guilford Press.

Markley, R. P., Zelhart, P. F., & Jackson, T. T. (Eds.). (1982). *Explorations with fixed-role therapy: First studies by students of George A. Kelly*. Fort Hays State University. https://doi.org/10.58809/SAEZ9091

Marquis, A., & Douthit, K. (2006). The hegemony of "empirically supported treatment": Validating or violating? *Constructivism in the Human Sciences, 11*(1–2), 108–141.

Martínez-Delgado, A. (2002). Radical constructivism: Between realism and solipsism. *Science Education, 86*(6), 840–855. https://doi.org/10.1002/sce.10005

Matos, M., Santos, A., Gonçalves, M., & Martins, C. (2009). Innovative moments and change in narrative therapy. *Psychotherapy Research, 19*(1), 68–80. https://doi.org/10.1080/10503300802430657

Maturana, H. R., & Varela, F. J. (1992). *The tree of knowledge: The biological roots of human understanding* (Rev. ed.; R. Paolucci, Trans.). Shambhala.

McCrae, R. R. (2017). The five-factor model across cultures. In A. T. Church (Ed.), *The Praeger handbook of personality across cultures: Trait psychology across cultures* (pp. 47–71). Praeger/ABC-CLIO.

McCrae, R. R., & Costa, P. T., Jr. (1997). Personality trait structure as a human universal. *American Psychologist, 52*(5), 509–516. https://doi.org/10.1037/0003-066X.52.5.509

McCrae, R. R., & John, O. P. (1992). An introduction to the five-factor model and its applications. *Journal of Personality, 60*(2), 175–215. https://doi.org/10.1111/j.1467-6494.1992.tb00970.x

McGuinty, E. F., Bird, B. M., Silva, J. R., Morrow, D. K., & Armstrong, D. C. (2018). Externalizing metaphors therapy and innovative moments: A four-session treatment group for anxiety. *International Journal of Group Psychotherapy, 68*(3), 428–457. https://doi.org/10.1080/00207284.2018.1429926

McNamee, S., Rasera, E. F., & Martins, P. (2023). *Practicing therapy as social construction.* SAGE Publishing.

McWilliams, S. A. (2016a). Cultivating constructivism: Inspiring intuition and promoting process and pragmatism. *Journal of Constructivist Psychology, 29*(1), 1–29. https://doi.org/10.1080/10720537.2014.980871

McWilliams, S. A. (2016b). Personal construct psychology and Buddhism. In D. A. Winter & N. Reed (Eds.), *The Wiley handbook of personal construct psychology* (pp. 439–451). John Wiley & Sons. https://doi.org/10.1002/9781118508275.ch35

McWilliams, S. A. (2022). Truth as trophy: The social construction of veracity. *Journal of Constructivist Psychology, 35*(2), 448–459. https://doi.org/10.1080/10720537.2020.1727386

Menand, L. (2001). *The metaphysical club: A story of ideas in America.* Farrar, Straus and Giroux.

Mende, F., Batista, J., O'Keeffe, S., Midgley, N., Braga, R., Gonçalves, M. M., & Henriques, M. R. (2024). Innovative moments with young patients treated for depression: An analysis of post-therapy interviews. *Clinical Psychology & Psychotherapy, 31*(1), Article e2896. https://doi.org/10.1002/cpp.2896

Metcalfe, C., Winter, D., & Viney, L. (2007). The effectiveness of personal construct psychotherapy in clinical practice: A systematic review and meta-analysis. *Psychotherapy Research, 17*(4), 431–442. https://doi.org/10.1080/10503300600755115

Michaels, L. (2020, March 24). *Therapy that sticks. Aeon.* https://aeon.co/essays/why-depth-therapy-is-more-enduring-than-a-quick-fix-of-cbt

Minuchin, S. (1974). *Families and family therapy.* Harvard University Press. https://doi.org/10.4159/9780674041127

Mitchell, G. (n.d.). *Bertalanffy's general systems theory.* https://trans4mind.com/mind-development/systems.html

Monk, G., Winslade, J., Crocket, K., & Epston, D. (1997). *Narrative therapy in practice: The archaeology of hope.* Jossey-Bass.

Monk, G., & Zamani, N. (2019). Narrative therapy and the affective turn: Part I. *Journal of Systemic Therapies, 38*(2), 1–19. https://doi.org/10.1521/jsyt.2019.38.2.1

Montesano, A., Oliveira, J. T., & Gonçalves, M. M. (2017). How do self-narratives change during psychotherapy? A review of innovative moments research. *Journal of Systemic Therapies, 36*(3), 81–96. https://doi.org/10.1521/jsyt.2017.36.3.81

Nagizadeh-Alamdari, M., & Smkhani-Akbarinejhad, H. (2022). Effectiveness of narrative therapy on body dysmorphic concern & perceived self-efficacy of female students with obesity & overweight. *The Journal of Psychology, 26*(2), 182–189.

Nasim, R., Shimshi, S., Ziv-Beiman, S., Peri, T., Fernández-Navarro, P., Oliveira, J. T., & Gonçalves, M. M. (2019). Exploring innovative moments in a brief integrative psychotherapy case study. *Journal of Psychotherapy Integration, 29*(4), 359–373. https://doi.org/10.1037/int0000148

Nasim, R. S., Ziv-Beiman, S., Leibovich, A., Sousa, I., Gonçalves, M. M., & Peri, T. (2021). Innovative moments and session impact in brief integrative psychotherapy: An exploratory study. *Journal of Psychotherapy Integration, 31*(1), 86–103. https://doi.org/10.1037/int0000189

Neimeyer, R. A. (1995). Limits and lessons of constructivism: Some critical reflections. *Journal of Constructivist Psychology, 8*(4), 339–361. https://doi.org/10.1080/10720539508405914

Neimeyer, R. A. (1997). Problems and prospects in constructivist psychotherapy. *Journal of Constructivist Psychology, 10*(1), 51–74. https://doi.org/10.1080/10720539708404611

Neimeyer, R. A., & Mahoney, M. J. (Eds.). (1995). *Constructivism in psychotherapy.* American Psychological Association. https://doi.org/10.1037/10170-000

Neimeyer, R. A., & Raskin, J. D. (2000). On practicing postmodern therapy in modern times. In R. A. Neimeyer & J. D. Raskin (Eds.), *Constructions of disorder: Meaning-making frameworks for psychotherapy* (pp. 3–14). American Psychological Association. https://doi.org/10.1037/10368-001

REFERENCES

Neimeyer, R. A., & Raskin, J. D. (2001). Varieties of constructivism in psychotherapy. In K. S. Dobson (Ed.), *Handbook of cognitive–behavioral therapies* (2nd ed., pp. 393–430). The Guilford Press.

Oates, J. C. (1999, December 30). The calendar's new clothes. *The New York Times*. https://www.nytimes.com/1999/12/30/opinion/the-calendar-s-new-clothes.html

Paris, M. E., & Epting, F. R. (2015). Dewey between the lines: George Kelly and the pragmatist tradition. *Journal of Constructivist Psychology, 28*(2), 181–189. https://doi.org/10.1080/10720537.2014.943915

Pavlović, J. (2011). Personal construct psychology and social constructionism are not incompatible: Implications of a reframing. *Theory & Psychology, 21*(3), 396–411. https://doi.org/10.1177/0959354310380302

Paz, C., Aguilera, M., Salla, M., Compañ, V., Medina, J. C., Bados, A., García-Grau, E., Castel, A., Cañete Crespillo, J., Montesano, A., Medeiros-Ferreira, L., & Feixas, G. (2020). Personal construct therapy vs cognitive behavioral therapy in the treatment of depression in women with fibromyalgia: Study protocol for a multicenter randomized controlled trial. *Neuropsychiatric Disease and Treatment, 16*, 301–311. https://doi.org/10.2147/NDT.S235161

Paz, C., Pucurull, O., & Feixas, G. (2016). Change in symptoms and personal construct structure in anxiety disorders: A preliminary study on the effects of constructivist therapy. *Journal of Constructivist Psychology, 29*(3), 231–247. https://doi.org/10.1080/10720537.2014.943914

Pepper, S. C. (1970). *World hypotheses: A study in evidence*. University of California Press. https://doi.org/10.1525/9780520341869 (Original work published 1942)

Piazza-Bonin, E., Neimeyer, R. A., Alves, D., & Smigelsky, M. (2016). Innovative moments in humanistic therapy II: Analysis of change processes across the course of three cases of grief therapy. *Journal of Constructivist Psychology, 29*(3), 298–317. https://doi.org/10.1080/10720537.2015.1118713

Piazza-Bonin, E., Neimeyer, R. A., Alves, D., Smigelsky, M., & Crunk, E. (2016). Innovative moments in humanistic therapy I: Process and outcome of eminent psychotherapists working with bereaved clients. *Journal of Constructivist Psychology, 29*(3), 269–297. https://doi.org/10.1080/10720537.2015.1118712

Pinheiro, R. T., Botella, L., de Avila Quevedo, L., Pinheiro, K. A. T., Jansen, K., Osório, C. M., Herrero, O., da Silva Magalhães, P. O. V., Farias, A. D., & da Silva, R. A. (2014). Maintenance of the effects of cognitive behavioral and relational constructivist psychotherapies in the treatment of women with postpartum depression: A randomized clinical trial. *Journal of Constructivist Psychology, 27*(1), 59–68. https://doi.org/10.1080/10720537.2013.814093

Porter, C. (Composer). (1934). *Anything goes* [Musical]. Directed by Howard Lindsay, performance by Ethel Merman, William Gaxton, and Victor Moore,

November 21, 1934, Alvin Theater, New York City. https://playbill.com/production/anything-goes-alvin-theatre-vault-0000000954

Priebe, S. (2021). Patients in mental healthcare should be referred to as patients and not service users. *BJPsych Bulletin, 45*(6), 327–328. https://doi.org/10.1192/bjb.2021.40

Procter, H., & Winter, D. A. (2020). *Personal and relational construct psychotherapy*. Palgrave Macmillan. https://doi.org/10.1007/978-3-030-52177-6

Rajalakshmi, N. (2023, October 4). What colors do dogs see? Scientific American. https://www.scientificamerican.com/article/what-colors-do-dogs-see/

Rani, A., Raman, K. J., Antony, S., Ammapattian, T., & Chethan, B. (2024). Narrative therapy with Dalit female survivors of violence. *Violence and Gender, 11*(1), 53–57. https://doi.org/10.1089/vio.2023.0026

Raskin, J. D. (1999). Metaphors and meaning: Constructing the creative psychotherapist. *Journal of Constructivist Psychology, 12*(4), 331–347. https://doi.org/10.1080/107205399266046

Raskin, J. D. (2001). On relativism in constructivist psychology. *Journal of Constructivist Psychology, 14*(4), 285–313. https://doi.org/10.1080/10720530126044

Raskin, J. D. (2002). Constructivism in psychology: Personal construct psychology, radical constructivism, and social constructionism. *American Communication Journal, 5*(3). https://ac-journal.org/journal/vol5/iss3/special/raskin.pdf

Raskin, J. D. (2007). Assimilative integration in constructivist psychotherapy. *Journal of Psychotherapy Integration, 17*(1), 50–69. https://doi.org/10.1037/1053-0479.17.1.50

Raskin, J. D. (2011). On essences in constructivist psychology. *Journal of Theoretical and Philosophical Psychology, 31*(4), 223–239. https://doi.org/10.1037/a0025006

Raskin, J. D. (2015). An introductory perturbation: What is constructivism and is there a future in it? In J. D. Raskin, S. K. Bridges, & J. S. Kahn (Eds.), *Studies in meaning 5: Perturbing the status quo in constructivist psychology* (pp. 3–27). Pace University Press.

Raskin, J. D. (2023). Using context-centered and person-centered therapies to unite a divided nation. *The Humanistic Psychologist, 51*(1), 2–14. https://doi.org/10.1037/hum0000276

Raskin, J. D., & Bridges, S. K. (2024). Constructivist theories in psychotherapy. In F. T. L. Leong, J. L. Callahan, J. Zimmerman, M. J. Constantino, & C. F. Eubanks (Eds.), *APA handbook of psychotherapy: Vol. 1. Theory-driven practice and disorder-driven practice* (pp. 257–272). American Psychological Association. https://doi.org/10.1037/0000353-015

Raskin, J. D., Bridges, S. K., & Kahn, J. S. (2015). Constructivism: Where do we go from here? In J. D. Raskin, S. K. Bridges, & J. S. Kahn (Eds.), *Studies in meaning 5: Perturbing the status quo in constructivist psychology* (pp. 300–325). Pace University Press.

Raskin, J. D., & Debany, A. E. (2018). The inescapability of ethics and the impossibility of "anything goes": A constructivist model of ethical meaning-making. *Journal of Constructivist Psychology, 31*(4), 343–360. https://doi.org/10.1080/10720537.2017.1383954 (Reprinted from *Ethics in action: Dialogue between knowledge and practice*, pp. 13–32, by S. Cipolletta & E. Gius, Eds., 2012, LED)

Raskin, J. D., & Efran, J. S. (2020). The practice of context-centered therapy: A conversation with Jay S. Efran. *The Humanistic Psychologist, 48*(2), 202–219. https://doi.org/10.1037/hum0000143

Raskin, J. D., & Efran, J. S. (2021). The coronavirus in context: Guidance for psychotherapists during a pandemic. *Journal of Humanistic Psychology, 61*(2), 160–172. https://doi.org/10.1177/0022167820937509

Raskin, J. D., & Epting, F. R. (1993). Personal construct theory and the argument against mental illness. *International Journal of Personal Construct Psychology, 6*(4), 351–369. https://doi.org/10.1080/08936039308405629

Raskin, J. D., & Lewandowski, A. M. (2000). The construction of disorder as human enterprise. In R. A. Neimeyer & J. D. Raskin (Eds.), *Constructions of disorder: Meaning-making frameworks for psychotherapy* (pp. 15–40). American Psychological Association. https://doi.org/10.1037/10368-002

Raskin, J. D., & Morano, L. A. (2004). Credulous approach. In J. Scheer & B. Walker (Eds.), *The internet encyclopaedia of personal construct psychology.* http://www.pcp-net.org/encyclopaedia/cred-appr.html

Raskin, J. D., Weihs, K. D., & Morano, L. A. (2005). Personal construct psychotherapy meets constructivism: Convergence, divergence, and possibility. In D. A. Winter & L. L. Viney (Eds.), *Advances in personal construct psychotherapy* (pp. 3–20). Whurr Publishers. https://doi.org/10.1002/9780470713686.ch1

Rogers, C. R. (1951). *Client-centered therapy.* Constable.

Rogers, C. R. (1959). A theory of therapy, personality, and interpersonal relationships, as developed in the client-centered framework. In S. Koch (Ed.), *Psychology: A study of science: Vol. 3. Formulations of the person and the social contact* (pp. 184–256). McGraw-Hill.

Salas Llanas, I. (2018). Brevísimo análisis doxográfico sobre el Constructivismo: de los presocráticos a la cibernética de segundo orden [A (very) brief doxographical analysis of constructivism: From pre-Socratics to second-order cybernetics]. *Bajo Palabra, 18*, 61–76. https://doi.org/10.15366/bp2018.18.003

Santos, A., Gonçalves, M. M., & Matos, M. (2011). Innovative moments and poor outcome in narrative therapy. *Counselling & Psychotherapy Research, 11*(2), 129–139. https://doi.org/10.1080/14733140903398153

REFERENCES

Shapiro, D. A., Barkham, M., Stiles, W. B., Hardy, G. E., Rees, A., Reynolds, S., & Startup, M. (2003). Time is of the essence: A selective review of the fall and rise of brief therapy research. *Psychology and Psychotherapy: Theory, Research and Practice, 76*(3), 211–235. https://doi.org/10.1348/147608303322362460

Sheehan, M. J. (1985). A personal construct study of depression. *The British Journal of Medical Psychology, 58*(2), 119–128. https://doi.org/10.1111/j.2044-8341.1985.tb02624.x

Sheena, L., Kivity, Y., Shimshi, S., Tuval-Mashiach, R., & Peri, T. (2024). How does change occur in psychotherapy? Innovative moments predict stronger therapeutic alliance and functional improvement in a psychodynamic case study. *Journal of Constructivist Psychology, 37*(1), 7–20. https://doi.org/10.1080/10720537.2023.2248529

Shotter, J. (1995). In dialogue: Social construction and radical constructivism. In L. P. Steffe & J. Gale (Eds.), *Constructivism in education* (pp. 41–56). Lawrence Erlbaum Associates.

Slife, B. D., Yanchar, S. C., & Williams, B. (1999). Conceptions of determinism in radical behaviorism: A taxonomy. *Behavior and Philosophy, 27*(2), 75–96.

Smothermon, R. (1980). *Winning through enlightenment*. Context Publications.

Spektor, B. (2023, January 31). This is why Japan has blue traffic lights instead of green. *Reader's Digest*. https://www.rd.com/article/heres-japan-blue-traffic-lights/

Steffe, L. P., & Kieren, T. (1994). Radical constructivism and mathematics education. *Journal for Research in Mathematics Education, 25*(6), 711–733. https://doi.org/10.2307/749582

Steinglass, P. (1984). Family systems theory and therapy: A clinical application of general systems theory. *Psychiatric Annals, 14*(8), 582–586. https://doi.org/10.3928/0048-5713-19840801-09

Stewart, A. E., & Barry, J. R. (1991). Origins of George Kelly's constructivism in the work of Korzybski and Moreno. *International Journal of Personal Construct Psychology, 4*(2), 121–136. https://doi.org/10.1080/08936039108404768

Stewart, T., & Birdsall, M. (2001). A review of the contribution of personal construct psychology to stammering therapy. *Journal of Constructivist Psychology, 14*(3), 215–226. https://doi.org/10.1080/10720530151143557

Stoll, T. (2020). Hans Vaihinger. In E. N. Zalta (Ed.), *The Stanford encyclopedia of philosophy* (Spring 2020). Stanford University. https://plato.stanford.edu/archives/spr2020/entries/vaihinger/

Sun, L., Liu, X., Weng, X., Deng, H., Li, Q., Liu, J., & Luan, X. (2022). Narrative therapy to relieve stigma in oral cancer patients: A randomized controlled trial. *International Journal of Nursing Practice, 28*(4), Article e12926. https://doi.org/10.1111/ijn.12926

Teasdale, J. D. (2004). Mindfulness-based cognitive therapy. In J. Yiend (Ed.), *Cognition, emotion and psychopathology: Theoretical, empirical and clinical directions* (pp. 270–289). Cambridge University Press. https://doi.org/10.1017/CBO9780511521263.015

Thomson, J. (2023, April 9). The species that change sex. *Newsweek.* https://www.newsweek.com/animals-change-sex-hermaphrodite-evolution-1793036

Tomm, K. (1989). Externalizing the problem and internalizing personal agency. *Journal of Strategic & Systemic Therapies, 8*(1), 54–59. https://doi.org/10.1521/jsst.1989.8.1.54

Tschudi, F. (1977). Loaded and honest questions: A construct theory view of symptoms and therapy. In D. Bannister (Ed.), *New perspectives in personal construct theory* (pp. 321–350). Academic Press.

Vaihinger, H. (1935). *The philosophy of "as if": A system of the theoretical, practical and religious fictions of mankind* (2nd ed.; C. K. Ogden, Trans.). Kegan Paul, Trench, Trubner & Co. https://archive.org/details/in.ernet.dli.2015.188061 (Original work published 1911)

Vasquez, M. J. T., & Johnson, J. D. (2022). *Multicultural therapy: A practice imperative.* American Psychological Association. https://doi.org/10.1037/0000279-000

Velton, E. (Ed.). (2007). *Under the influence: Reflections of Albert Ellis in the work of others.* Sharp Press.

Vico, G. (1948). *The new science of Giambattista Vico* (3rd ed.; T. G. Bergin & M. H. Fisch, Trans.). Cornell University Press. (Original work published 1744)

Vico, G. (1988). *On the most ancient wisdom of the Italians: Unearthed from the origins of the Latin language* (L. M. Palmer, Ed. & Trans.). Cornell University Press. (Original work published 1710)

Viney, L. L. (1981). Experimenting with experience: A psychotherapeutic case study. *Psychotherapy: Theory, Research & Practice, 18*(2), 271–278. https://doi.org/10.1037/h0086090

Viney, L. L., Metcalfe, C., & Winter, D. A. (2006). The effectiveness of personal construct psychotherapy: A meta-analysis. In D. A. Winter & L. L. Viney (Eds.), *Personal construct psychotherapy: Advances in theory, practice and research* (pp. 347–364). Whurr Publishers.

Vromans, L. P., & Schweitzer, R. D. (2011). Narrative therapy for adults with major depressive disorder: Improved symptom and interpersonal outcomes. *Psychotherapy Research, 21*(1), 4–15. https://doi.org/10.1080/10503301003591792

Wampold, B. E., & Imel, Z. E. (2015). *The great psychotherapy debate: The evidence for what makes psychotherapy work* (2nd ed.). Routledge. https://doi.org/10.4324/9780203582015

Watson, S., & Winter, D. A. (2005). A process and outcome study of personal construct psychotherapy. In D. A. Winter & L. L. Viney (Eds.), *Personal construct psychotherapy: Advances in theory, practice and research* (pp. 335–346). Whurr Publishers. https://doi.org/10.1002/9780470713686.ch26

Watts, R. E. (2013, April). Reflecting "as if." *Counseling Today.* https://www.counseling.org/publications/counseling-today-magazine/article-archive/article/legacy/reflecting-as-if

Watts, R. E. (2017). Adlerian and constructivist therapies: A neo-Adlerian perspective. *Journal of Individual Psychology, 73*(2), 139–155. https://doi.org/10.1353/jip.2017.0012

White, M., & Epston, D. (1990). *Narrative means to therapeutic ends.* W.W. Norton & Company.

Wilchins, R. (2004). *Queer theory, gender theory: An instant primer.* Alyson Publications.

Will, H. (2018). The concept of the 50-minute hour: Time forming a frame for the unconscious. *International Forum of Psychoanalysis, 27*(1), 14–23. https://doi.org/10.1080/0803706X.2017.1372627

Winter, D. (2003). The evidence base for personal construct psychotherapy. In F. Fransella (Ed.), *International handbook of personal construct psychology* (pp. 265–272). John Wiley & Sons. https://doi.org/10.1002/0470013370.ch26

Winter, D., Gournay, K., Metcalfe, C., & Rossotti, N. (2006). Expanding agoraphobics' horizons: An investigation of the effectiveness of a personal construct psychotherapy intervention. *Journal of Constructivist Psychology, 19*(1), 1–29. https://doi.org/10.1080/10720530500311141

Winter, D., Sireling, L., Riley, T., Metcalfe, C., Quaite, A., & Bhandari, S. (2007). A controlled trial of personal construct psychotherapy for deliberate self-harm. *Psychology and Psychotherapy: Theory, Research and Practice, 80*(1), 23–37. https://doi.org/10.1348/147608306X102778

Winter, D. A. (1992). *Personal construct psychology in clinical practice: Theory, research and applications.* Routledge.

World Health Organization. (2019). *International statistical classification of diseases and related health problems* (11th ed.; 2022 release). https://icd.who.int/

Zelhart, P. F., & Jackson, T. T. (1983). George A. Kelly, 1931–1943: Environmental influences on a developing theorist. In J. Adams-Webber & J. C. Mancuso (Eds.), *Applications of personal construct theory* (pp. 137–154). Academic Press.

Index

Abandoned children, 94
ABC model, 51, 117
Abuse, sexual, 93
Action, concrete, 36
Active listening, 43
ADHD (attention-deficit/hyperactivity disorder), 95
Adler, Alfred, 16
Adolescents, 95
Aging, 94
Alternative constructions, 35, 45–46, 115
American Psychiatric Association, 23, 47, 85, 105–106
American Psychological Association, xii
Antirealism, 99–101
Anxiety, 43–44, 59, 64–65, 67, 69, 75, 80, 83, 94–95, 99
  social anxiety, 40, 93
"Anything goes" antirealism, 99–101
APA. *See* American Psychological Association
APA Dictionary of Psychology, xii
Appointment times, 86–87
Attention-deficit/hyperactivity disorder (ADHD), 95

Autism, 94
Awareness
  of contexts, 64
  of mind, 68–70

Baldwin, James Mark, 15
Bartlett, Frederick, 15
Behavior, 16–18, 94
  as an experiment, 17, 86, 114
  as an independent variable, 18
Behavior therapy, 18, 36
Being wrong, 68
Beliefs, "irrational," 44–45
Bereavement, 99
Berkeley, G., 11–12
Big Five personality model, 33, 105–106
Breast cancer survivors, 93
Brief-integrative therapies, 99
Brief therapy, 82–84
Buddhism, 10
Bulimia, 99

"The Calendar's New Clothes" (Oates), 3
Calkins, Mary Whiton, 15
Campbell, Donald, 15
Cancer, 93, 96

INDEX

Categories of understanding, 13
Cause and effect relationships, 12
CBT (cognitive behavior therapy),
   17, 44, 82, 93, 95, 98
Center for Studies in Cognitive
   Constructivist Psychotherapy,
   108
Changing contexts, difficulty of, 88–89
Children, 94
China, ancient, 10–11
Clapton, Eric, 111–115
Client, role of, 37–39
Client complaints, elaboration of,
   44–45
Cognitive and social therapy, 108
Cognitive schemas, 59
Cognitive therapies, 18–20, 108
Coherence, 59–61
Coherence Psychology Institute, 109
Coherence therapy, 59, 96, 117
Colors, as symbols, 4
Concrete action, 36
Conditioning, 18
Confiding relationship, 41
Constructions, alternative, 45–46
Constructive alternativism, 22, 117
Constructive ideas in psychotherapy,
   16–20
Constructive psychology, integrated,
   28–34, 119
Constructive theories, 6, 117
Constructive therapies, 6–7, 117
   cognitive therapies, vs., 19
   evidence base for efficacy of, 91–99
   future directions for, 103–109
   objections to, 93, 99–102
   terminology, 34, 102
   training opportunities, 108–109
Construing, 19–20, 101. *See also*
   epistemological construing
   and ontological construing
Context-centered therapy, 61–65, 97,
   107, 117

Contexts, 118
   awareness of, 64
   changing, 88–89
   characteristics and examples of, 63
   cultural, 108
   digital nature of, 62–63
   shifting, 61–65
Contextualism, 104, 106–108, 118
Contiguity, 12
Cooley, Charles H., 15
Core constructs, 48, 118
Countertransference, 57
Coventry Constructivist Centre (U.K.),
   109
Credulous approach, 43–47, 118
Credulous listening, 43, 46–47
Cultural context, 108

Delusional behavior, 94
Dependent variables, 18
Depersonalizing life, 65, 70–73
Depression, 43, 93, 70, 80, 93, 97, 99
Dewey, John, 15, 17
*Diagnostic and Statistical Manual of
   Mental Disorders* (*DSM-5-TR*;
   American Psychiatric Asso-
   ciation), 47, 85, 105
Digital nature of contexts, 62–63
Discourses, 26–27, 37, 74, 118
Discourse user, person as, 38–40
Distress, myths of, 41
Dulwich Center, 109

Early psychology, 14–16
Eating disorders, 47, 93, 96, 99
ECPE (empirically confirmed process
   of erasure), 96, 118
Effectiveness, of constructive thera-
   pies, 91–99
Efran, Jay, 36, 62, 86
Ego strength, 80
Einstein, Albert, 91
Elements, of psychotherapy, 41–42

152

INDEX

Element sets, 47–48
Emotional learnings, 59
Emotional skills, 94
Empirically confirmed process of erasure (ECPE), 96, 118
Epistemological construing, 32–33, 101, 118
Epistobabble, 101–102, 118
Erasure, empirically confirmed process of, 96, 118
Evaluation, constructive therapies, 91–102
   criticisms, 99–102
   efficacy, 92–99
Evidence base for effectiveness of constructive therapies, 91–99
Exceptions, 76–77, 118. *See also* innovative moments, sparkling moments, and unique outcomes
Experiential personal construct theory, 118
Experiential personal construct therapy, 54–57
Externalizing the problem, 75–77, 118
Eyes, human, 4–5

Faith, in healing relationship, 41
Fallacies, nominal, 79–81, 121
Female-male dichotomy, 5–6
Fixed roles, 52–54
Fixed-role sketches, 54–55, 118–119
Fixed-role therapy, 17, 52–54, 93–94, 119
Forensic clients, 93
Formism, 104–106, 119
Four premises of an integrated constructive psychology, 119
Frameworks, 113
Frank, Jerome, 41

Gaps, 77–79, 119
Gender roles, 5–6
General semantics, 17
Gestalt psychology, 15

Glasersfeld, E. von, 11, 21
Gorgias, 10
Great Depression, 17
Greece, ancient, 10–11
Grid
   implications, 51
   repertory (rep), 47–49, 122
   resistance to change, 51, 122
Grief and grief therapy, 99, 109
Group therapies, 99

Hayek, Frederick, 15
Healing relationships, 41
Healing rituals, 41–42
Helmholtz, Hermann von, 14
Heraclitus, 10, 114
History, constructive theories, 9–20
   ancient Greece and China, 10–11
   constructive ideas in psychotherapy, 16–20
   early psychology, 14–16
   Locke, Berkeley, and Hume, 11–12
   Vico, Kant, and Vaihinger, 12–14
Hoyt, M. F., 7
Humanistic therapies, 98
Hume, David, 11–14

ICD-11 (*International Classification of Diseases and Related Health Problems*, 11th ed.; WHO), 105
IM (innovative moments), 97–99, 119–120. *See also* exceptions, sparkling moments, and unique outcomes
IMCS (innovative moments coding system), 97–98, 120
Implications grid, 51, 119
Independent variables, 18
Indicative mood, 115, 119
Infeld, Leopold, 91
Informational closure, 28
Informationally closed system, 25, 28–29, 31, 119

Innovative moments (IM), 97–99, 119–120. *See also* exceptions, sparkling moments, and unique outcomes
Institute of Constructivist Psychotherapy (Padua, Italy), 108
Integrated constructive psychology, 28–34, 119
Interaction, orthogonal, 65–67, 121
International Classification of Diseases and Related Health Problems (11th ed.; *ICD-11*; WHO), 105
Intersubjective reality, 31, 120
Invitational mood, 115, 120
"Irrational" beliefs, 44–45

James, William, 15
Juvenile boot camp, adolescents in, 95

Kant, Immanuel, 12–14
Kelly, George
   on construing, 101
   on credulous approach, 43
   on experience, 103
   and fixed-role therapy, 16–19, 93
   on invitational mood, 115
   on reifying ideas, 10–11, 113
   on therapy process, 35–38
Korzybski, Alfred, 7, 17

Laddering, 48, 50–51, 120
Language, 22, 36–37, 39, 64, 80–81, 85, 87
   and indicative mood, 119
   living in, 15
   philology and, 40–41
   and the reification of ideas, 112-113
   understanding as constituted through, 31
Lao Tzu, 10
Learnings, emotional, 59
Leitner, Larry, 54–55
Life, depersonalizing, 70–73

Listening, 43, 46–47
Locke, John, 11–12
Long-term therapy, 82–84
Lorenz, Konrad, 15

Macrosocial processes, 74, 81–82, 120
Mahoney, Michael J., 7, 9
Male-female dichotomy, 5–6
Manifold, 13
Mapping personal constructs, 47–51
Mapping the influence of the problem, 76, 120
Mead, George Herbert, 15
Meaning, of words, 21
Meaning-making, 8, 25, 28, 29, 30–31, 38, 42, 51, 54–55, 59, 73, 85, 101, 106, 112
Meaning reconstruction, 99
Mechanism, 104–106, 120
Medical model, 37, 41, 84–85, 92, 106
Methodological pluralism, 92
Microsocial processes, 74, 81–82, 120
Mind, 11–13, 15
   in context-centered therapy, 65, 68–71, 83–84, 120–121
Mood disorders, 95
Mood problems, 93
Moreno, 17
Myths, of distress, 41

Narratives, 75–77, 99
Narrative solutions therapy, 77–79, 97, 121
Narrative therapy, 75–77, 94–96, 109, 121
Narrative Therapy Initiative, 109
Neimeyer, Robert, 102
Nominal fallacies, 79–81, 121
Noumena, 13

Oates, Joyce Carol, 3–5
Obstacles, to therapy processes, 84–89

INDEX

Ontological construing, 32–33, 100–101, 121
Opposite-meaning words, 21
Optimal therapeutic distance, 57, 121
Oral cancer, 96
Organicism, 106–108, 121
Original learnings, 59
Orphaned children, 94
Orthogonal interaction, 65–67, 69, 89, 115, 121

Paraphilias, 93
Past, as privileged, 85–86
Pepper, S. C., 104–108
Person
    as discourse user, 38–39, 121
    as philological consultant, 40–41
    as research collaborator, 39–40
    as scientist, 37–38, 121
Person-centered therapy, 43, 77
Personal constructivism, 21, 22–24, 28, 30, 122
Personal constructs, 22, 23, 42–43, 47–51, 121
    mapping, 47–51
    revising, 42–43
    subordinate/superordinate, 48, 50–51
Personal construct therapy, 23–24, 34, 42–43, 59, 65, 77, 93–94, 108, 121–122. *See also* fixed-role therapy
    assessment in, 47
    experiential personal construct therapy, 54–57
Persuasion and Healing (Frank), 41
Phenomena, 13
Philological consultant, 39, 40–41, 84, 122
Philology, 40–41
Phobias, social, 94–95
Photoreceptors, 4–5
Physical problems, 94

Piaget, Jean, 15
Pierce, Charles, 15
Portland Institute for Loss and Transition, 109
Postmodern therapies. *See* constructive therapies
Pragmatism, 15, 17, 111, 113
Preferred view, 77–78, 122
Premises, of integrated constructive psychology, 28–34, 119
Pre-Socratic thinkers, 10
Preverbal construing, 56, 63, 122
Primary qualities, 11–12
Problematic self-narratives, 98
Problems
    externalizing, 75–77, 118
    mapping the influence of, 76
Problem-saturated stories, 75, 122
Protagoras, 10
Psychodrama, 17
Psychodynamic therapy, 56, 82, 91, 93, 98
Psychology, early, 14–16
Psychosis, 93, 94
Psychotherapy, elements of, 41–42
Pyramiding, 51, 122

Qualities, primary and secondary, 11–12

Radical constructivism, 11, 13, 21, 24–26, 28, 30, 114, 122
Rationale, of distress, 41
Reality, intersubjective, 31, 120
Reality correspondence, 19
Reciprocal determinism, 107, 122
Reconstruing, 22, 35, 100
    and externalizing, 77
    and innovative moments (IMs), 98-99
Reifying, of ideas, 5–6, 7, 10–11, 74, 112–113
Relations, interpersonal, 55

INDEX

Relationship(s), 29, 32, 44, 50, 74, 101, 112
  cause and effect, 12
  confiding, 41
  healing, 41
  role, 43, 54–58, 123
  skills, 94
  social constructionism and, 26
  therapist-client, 41–42
Repertory (rep) grid, 47–49, 106, 122
Research collaboration, 39–40
Resemblance, 12
Resistance to change grid, 51, 122
Revising personal constructs, 42–43
Rituals, for healing, 41–42
Role relationships, 54–58, 123
Role(s)
  of the client, 36, 37–39
  fixed. *See* fixed roles
  gender, 5–6
  of therapist, 36, 39–41
Role therapy, 17. *See also* fixed-role therapy
Root metaphor theory, 123

Saussure, Ferdinand de, 15
School of Constructivist Psychotherapy (Padua, Italy), 108
Scientist, person as, 37–38, 121
Secondary qualities, 11–12
Self, 47, 55, 66, 77
  in context-centered therapy, 65, 68–71, 77–78, 83–84, 123
Self-awareness, 68–70
Self-characterization, 52. *See also* fixed-role therapy
Self-esteem, 7, 27, 80
Self-harm, 26, 93
Self-narratives, 75
  problematic, 98
Self-pathologizing, 67
Self-understanding, 82
Semantics, general, 17

Session duration, 86
Sex dichotomy, 5–6
Sexual abuse, 93
Sexual functioning, in women with skin cancer, 96
Sexual violence, trauma of, 96
Shifting contexts, 61–65
Sketches, fixed-role, 52–54, 118–119
Skills, 94
Skin cancer, sexual functioning in women with, 96
Social and emotional skills, children's, 94
Social anxiety, 40, 93
Social beings, 31–32
Social constructionism, 15, 21, 26–27, 28, 31, 73–74, 109, 114, 123
Social phobias, 94–95
Social skills, 94
Solution-focused therapy, 77
Sparkling moments, 76, 97, 123. *See also* exceptions, innovative moments, and unique outcomes
Stigma, of oral cancer, 96
Stories, 6, 64, 73–74, 75–76, 85, 97, 114
Strategic therapy, 77
Stress, 94
Structure determinism, 24–26, 123
Stuttering, 93
Subordinate/superordinate personal constructs, 48, 50–51

Taos Institute (New Mexico), 109
Termination, of therapy, 87–88
Theories, 21–34
  integrated constructive psychology, 28–34
  personal constructivism, 22–24
  radical constructivism, 24–26
  social constructionism, 26–27
Therapeutic distance, optimal, 57, 121
Therapist, role of, 39–41

INDEX

Therapist-client relationship, 41–42
Therapy, long-term, 82–84
Therapy length, 86
Therapy process, 35–89
    adopting a credulous approach, 43–47, 118
    brief vs. long-term, 82–84
    depersonalizing life, 70–73
    encouraging awareness of mind and self, 68–70
    externalizing the problem, 75–77, 118
    fostering coherence, 59–61
    having clients enact fixed roles, 52–54
    identifying nominal fallacies, 79–81, 121
    mapping personal constructs, 47–51
    microsocial and macrosocial processes, 81–82, 120
    narrative solutions therapy, 77–79, 97, 121
    obstacles, 84–89
    orthogonal interaction, 65–67, 121
    revising personal constructs, 42–43
    revising stories together, 73–74
    role of the client, 37–39
    role of the therapist, 39–41
    role of the therapist-client relationship, 41–42
    shifting contexts, 61–65
    working interpersonally using role relationships, 54–58
Training opportunities, 108–109
Transdiagnostic therapies, 99
Transference, 56
Trauma, 66, 94, 96

Understanding
    categories of, 13
    ways of, 59
Unique outcomes, 76, 97, 119. *See also* exceptions, innovative moments, and sparkling moments
University of Barcelona, 108
University of Hertfordshire, 108
University of Melbourne, 109
University of Padua, 108

Vaihinger, Hans, 14, 16
Validity, 15
Vancouver School for Narrative Therapy, 109
Variables, dependent and independent, 18
Viability, 15
Vico, Giambattista, 12–14

Ways of understanding the world, 59
WHO (World Health Organization), 105
Whorf, Benjamin, 15
Women, with skin cancer, sexual functioning in, 96
Word meaning, 21
Working interpersonally, 54–58
World Health Organization (WHO), 105
Wundt, Wilhelm, 14

Xenophanes, 10

About the Author

Jonathan D. Raskin, PhD, earned his bachelor of arts degree in psychology from Vassar College and his PhD in counseling psychology from the University of Florida. He is a professor of psychology and counselor education at the State University of New York at New Paltz, where he currently serves as interim associate provost for academic advising. Raskin is a licensed psychologist with an active private practice.

In addition to his many journal articles and book chapters on constructive therapies, Raskin is author of *Psychopathology and Mental Distress: Contrasting Perspectives* (2nd ed.), which was selected by the Association of College & Research Libraries' *Choice* publication as one of its 2024 outstanding academic titles. In 2020–2021, Raskin served as president of the Society for Humanistic Psychology (Division 32 of the American Psychological Association). He previously served as coeditor of the *Journal of Constructivist Psychology*.

About the Series Editor

Matt Englar-Carlson, PhD, is a professor and chair of Department of Counselor and the director of the Center for Boys and Men at California State University, Fullerton. A Fellow of the American Psychological Association, Dr. Englar-Carlson's scholarship focuses on training helping professionals to work more effectively with boys and men across the full range of human diversity, social justice and diversity issues in psychological training and practice, and theories of psychotherapy. Dr. Englar-Carlson coedited the books *In the Room with Men: A Casebook of Therapeutic Change, Counseling Troubled Boys: A Guidebook for Professionals, Beyond the 50-Minute Hour: Therapists Involved in Meaningful Social Action,* and *A Counselor's Guide to Working with Men,* and was featured in the APA-produced video *Engaging Men in Psychotherapy.* He was named Researcher of the Year, Professional of the Year, and received the Professional Service award by the Society for the Psychological Study of Men and Masculinities, and was one of the core authors of the *APA Guidelines for Professional Psychological Practice with Boys and Men.* He is the coauthor of *Adlerian Psychotherapy,* which is part of the Theories of Psychotherapy series. He is the clinical advisor for the men's mental health app, Mental, and serves on Movember's Global Men's Health Advisory Committee, and the advisory board for the Positive Masculinity Foundation.